THE WHICH? GUIDE TO
MANAGING ASTHMA

About the author

A pharmacologist by training, Mark Greener is now a medical journalist and editor, who has contributed to both consumer and specialist publications, including *Health Which?*. He has written widely on the subjects of drugs, nutrition and health for medical, nursing and consumer magazines, and is also the author of *The Which? Guide to Managing Stress. The Which? Guide to Managing Asthma* came about partly through his own experience of being an asthma sufferer.

Acknowledgements

The author and publishers would like to thank the National Asthma Campaign for their help in preparing this book.

THE WHICH? GUIDE TO MANAGING ASTHMA

MARK GREENER

CONSUMERS' ASSOCIATION

Which? Books are commissioned and researched by
Consumers' Association and published by
Which? Ltd, 2 Marylebone Road, London NW1 4DF
Email address: books@which.net

Distributed by The Penguin Group:
Penguin Books Ltd, 27 Wrights Lane, London W8 5TZ

First edition August 1997

British Library Cataloguing-in-Publication Data
A catalogue record for this book is available from the British Library

ISBN 0 85202 661 7

For a full list of Which? books, please write to
Which? Books, Castlemead, Gascoyne Way, Hertford X, SG14 1LH
or access our web site at http://www.which.net/

Cover design by Ridgeway Associates
Cover photograph by Damien Lovegrove/Science Photo Library
Illustrations by John Baxter
Typeset by Saxon Graphics Ltd, Derby
Printed and bound in Great Britain by Clays Ltd, St Ives plc

CONTENTS

★ Indicates that the addresses and telephone numbers will be found in the Addresses section starting on page 233

FOREWORD

About 150 million people worldwide suffer from asthma and nearly every survey shows that people want more information about their condition. Yet each person has a unique experience of asthma and different concerns and expectations.

The best place to elicit answers to these questions is within routine consultations with your doctor or nurse, but we all know how hurried such sessions may be – sometimes we may forget to ask the right questions, or in our preoccupation with asking the question forget the reply. This is where *The Which? Guide to Managing Asthma* comes in. It is aimed at everyone with asthma, containing a wealth of information capable of answering the most individual of queries.

Many people with asthma report that fear of an attack and uncertainty over a possible exacerbation are prime worries. Only when such concerns about the illness or its treatment are dispelled can sufferers begin to feel more comfortable about their situation. This book gives clear advice on how people can control their condition by themselves.

Armed with the information, both those with asthma and the parents of children with asthma will be able to enter into a proper partnership with their doctor or nurse to work together at controlling the condition and leading a full and active life.

Dr Martyn R. Partridge MD, FRCP,
Consultant Physician, Chest Clinic,
Whipps Cross Hospital, London,
Chief Medical Adviser to the National Asthma Campaign

INTRODUCTION

What do Ian Botham, Edwina Currie and the Olympic swimmer Adrian Moorhouse have in common? They, like one in ten adults in the UK today, have asthma.

Asthma is one of the commonest medical conditions in Britain. Four per cent of children below the age of three and ten per cent of 4- to 17-year-olds are now being treated for asthma. For a long time, asthma was the only preventable disease with an increasing death rate in the developed world. The British mortality rate of nearly 1,500 a year is still unacceptably high – although, compared to the number of sufferers, deaths from asthma are are rare.

Although asthma is often regarded as a modern scourge, blamed on our refined diet, pollution, smoking and the other hazards of twentieth-century life, it has always been with us. However, it is becoming more common. During the last decade the number of people consulting their GP about asthma has almost doubled and the number of working days lost to the disease increased by 55 per cent between 1991–2 and 1994–5. Meanwhile, many thousands of asthma sufferers endure daily symptoms that ruin their quality of life.

An increasing problem

Several factors can exacerbate the problem. For example, patients may not seek medical help and doctors may have difficulty diagnosing asthma in those patients who do because many other illnesses can mimic asthma. While childhood asthma gains most of the headlines – few sights are more distressing than a wheezing infant – asthma can strike for the first time at any age, even among elderly people. Indeed, deaths from asthma peak among the over-40s, yet many older people accept breathlessness as a sign of ageing and delay visiting their GP. Chapter 7 explores the problems of asthma in children/teenagers, adults and elderly people through commonly asked questions for each age group, while

Chapter 2 examines why diagnosing asthma can prove difficult and describes the tests for asthma used by doctors.

Many people find that poor air quality or chemicals in their work environment make breathing more difficult. Yet perhaps only a third of occupational asthma cases come to doctors' attention. *The Which? Guide to Managing Asthma* explores the factors that contribute to occupational asthma and investigates the role that triggers such as pollution play in exacerbating asthma. Though frequently at the mercy of pollen, the house dust mite and food allergies, asthma sufferers should not have to put up with poor quality of life. This book explains how you can take steps to avoid asthma triggers where possible and use effective treatments when this is not feasible. The book also makes suggestions about conquering nocturnal and exercise-induced asthma.

Are drugs the answer?

If you or your child have asthma, your first port of call should be your GP. GPs manage more than 90 per cent of people with asthma. Following the introduction of national guidelines in 1990 (most recently updated in February 1997), GPs' care of sufferers noticeably improved – and this is reflected in falling death rates. Asthma is also lucrative for pharmaceutical companies, so GPs are offered a wealth of industry-sponsored educational literature that further helps to raise awareness about asthma.

Despite this, the care that GPs offer still varies. A survey of neighbouring practices in Somerset, for example, revealed that diagnostic rates for asthma ranged from 2 to 12 per cent of the population, suggesting that doctors continue to under-diagnose and under-treat asthma. This book emphasises the importance of recognising the symptoms of asthma, acting on your concerns and presenting your GP with evidence that will aid diagnosis.

Modern drugs can be lifesavers as well as controlling symptoms from day to day. Prompt and effective treatment can prevent asthma developing from mild, reversible symptoms into a severe, entrenched problem. So it is important to watch for signs of asthma – this book tells you what to look for.

Asthma is caused by inflammation in the lungs. Treatment therefore aims to control the underlying inflammation with anti-inflammatories (preventers), usually inhaled steroids, while bronchodilators (relievers) – which open the airways – relieve acute symptoms. If the inflammation is effectively controlled you should need to use your bronchodilator once a day at the most. Chapter 5 takes a look at the risks and benefits of current asthma medication. Chapter 10 takes a look into the future and the possibilities of a cure for asthma.

Taking control

For it to be effective, patients need to take their medication as instructed. Yet despite the fact that they know they have a serious illness, they do not always do so – a problem known as non-compliance. One solution, Asthma Management Plans, which are personalised treatment guidelines, optimises patients' involvement. These plans rely on measurements of lung function (peak flow) that can detect an exacerbation before symptoms emerge.

Modern drugs allow most people with asthma to live normal, healthy lives. But despite these advances many asthma sufferers hold low expectations of treatment. Some adapt to, rather than eliminate, their symptoms. Some cannot come to terms with their condition, with the result that both they and their families experience high levels of stress.

Depression and anxiety can worsen asthma. However, there is no reason why people with asthma should suffer needlessly. Chapter 3 explores the mind–body link and the psychology of asthma in detail, explaining how to reduce the physical and psychological toll imposed by asthma. Complementary therapies, breathing exercises and relaxation techniques are among the solutions discussed in Chapter 9.

Despite the various obstacles to progress described above, most cases are mild and can be effectively and safely treated with modern drugs. For the moment, people with asthma should not rely on drugs alone: the many self-help measures described in this book can reduce the risk of an attack and help you live life to the full. You can take steps to control your asthma, rather than letting it control you. Read on and find out how.

CHAPTER 1

WHAT IS ASTHMA?

DESPITE being thought of as a modern scourge, asthma has always been with us. The earliest mention of the cluster of symptoms we now know of as asthma was made some 3,500 years ago in the Egyptian *Ebers Papyrus*. The word 'asthma' appears in Homer's *Iliad* in about the ninth century BC, where it means 'laboured breathing'. 'Asthma' was first used to describe the disease by the Greek physician Hippocrates who lived some 500 years later. However, the treatments for asthma concocted by Roman and Greek physicians, such as owls' blood in wine, owed more to magic than medicine.

The first book on asthma was written by the Spanish doctor Moses Maimonides while physician to the Sultan Saladin in AD 1190. Maimonides noted that asthma was characterised by sudden, unpredictable bouts of breathlessness. His treatments included copious amounts of hot chicken soup and sexual abstinence. He also advocated a holistic approach and had the humility to admit he lacked a 'magic cure' – something that still eludes us today.

Physicians in the seventeenth and eighteenth centuries recognised that asthma was due to constriction of the bronchi (the airways in the lung). One doctor called asthma the 'epilepsy of the lungs', reflecting the sudden and unpredictable nature of the attacks. However, today most people with asthma can detect when their symptoms are deteriorating and take steps to prevent a severe attack.

Throughout history, patients have taken a variety of folk remedies for the condition – some of which probably worked in the same way as today's bronchodilators. Yet it was not until the 1960s that doctors finally realised that asthma is an inflammatory disease. The immune systems of most people with asthma are exquisitely sensitive to minute amounts of triggers (such as pollen, cat fur or the house dust mite) that most people find innocuous. A growing understanding of the immune system's role in asthma triggered a revolution in treatment. Instead of just reversing the constriction, doctors now aim to control the underlying inflammation. As we head into the twenty-first century, doctors can prescribe a growing number of effective treatments that allow people with asthma to live fulfilled lives.

A growing problem

Asthma is never far from the headlines, reflecting the scale of the problem in the UK. Each year, over 1.8 million children and 7.2 million adults wheeze – one of asthma's hallmarks – while about 1.3 million children and 1.8 million adults (about 10–20 per cent of children and 5–10 per cent of adults) have diagnosed asthma. About two million people with asthma consult their GP every year; 95,000 need hospital treatment and 200,000 (one in ten adult asthma sufferers) are disabled by asthma.

Even these statistics underestimate the scale of the problem. Perhaps as many as seven per cent of the population have undiagnosed asthma, and asthma is becoming more common. In the UK, the number of people consulting their GP about asthma for the first time more than tripled over the last decade. The increase is even more marked among children – the number of 5- to 11-year-olds who experience asthma attacks increased threefold over the 1980s alone, while the number of children who wheeze occasionally increased by 60 per cent. Indeed, the number of British children who wheeze increased by 70 per cent between 1974 and 1986 – among 16-year-olds a rise from four to seven per cent.

Moreover, the increase is not confined to our polluted inner cities. Even in the Scottish Highlands, 14 per cent of 12-year-old children were diagnosed with asthma and a quarter were found to wheeze (about 89 per cent wheezed following a cold and 83 per cent after exercise). Some doctors predict that by the early years of the twenty-first century half of all people living in the UK will either wheeze or suffer from asthma before the age of 33.

The increase in wheezing confirms that the rising asthma rates are real. When doctors first noted the dramatic increase in cases, some suggested that the rise reflected an increase in awareness, with doctors being more likely to diagnose 'asthma' rather than labelling the disease as something else – 'wheezy bronchitis', for example. This may be partly true, but it is not the whole story. As we will see later, wheezing can be a symptom of a number of other conditions. Asthma does however account for a large proportion of wheezy lung diseases. Its increase cannot be merely written off as diagnostic fashion.

The effect on society

Despite doctors' increasing awareness, the death rate from asthma remains stubbornly high – although mortality has begun to decline in recent years. In 1995, 1,335 people died from asthma: about four people a day or one person every six hours. However, while childhood asthma grabs most of the headlines, deaths peak among middle-aged and elderly people. In 1994, 1,539 people over 45 died from asthma compared with 58 fatalities among those under 15 years of age. However, though children under 15 account for only two per cent of asthma deaths, they comprised almost half of the 94,700 admissions to hospital for asthma in 1995. The tragic irony is that specialists believe that better management could prevent 80 per cent of the deaths and at least 40 per cent of the hospital admissions.

Asthma exerts more than a human toll. Treating asthma costs the National Health Service about £473 million a year. The disease accounts for 11 million lost working days and two million lost school days. In 1995, asthma-related social security payments reached £70 million. In total, asthma costs the British economy over £1 billion a year.

So what is asthma? Why does it impose such as heavy human and economic toll? And what can you do to manage your or your child's asthma more effectively?

Inside our lungs

Unless something goes wrong, we do not really think about breathing. Each minute we take about 12 breaths, and, even at rest, about 7.5 litres of air move in and out of our lungs. Yet we live surrounded by a sea of pollutants, viruses and bacteria that hitch a lift on the airflow in and out of the lungs. Consequently, our lungs developed elaborate defences to protect the body from these airborne hazards. In asthma, these defence mechanisms seem to go wrong. To understand why, it is important to appreciate the lungs' normal role.

Physical structure

The **lungs** (see figure), which exchange toxic carbon dioxide for life-giving oxygen, are one of the largest organs in our bodies. Each lung weighs about 0.45kg, although as the left lung lies over the heart, the right lung is slightly larger. The right lung is made up of three lobes and the left lung of two lobes. Fully expanded, an adult's lungs hold about six litres of air.

Despite their size, the lungs are spongy and fragile, so they are encased in the bony ribcage and protected underneath by a thick muscular sheet, known as the **diaphragm**, which also plays an important role in **respiration** (breathing). Between each rib, a thick **intercostal muscle** aids breathing. Underneath the ribs, two membranes – the **pleura** – cover each lung and offer additional protection. These slide over each other when you breathe in (**inhale**) and out (**exhale**).

When you inhale, air moves in through your mouth and nose, then flows down through your throat and into the windpipe – also called the **trachea**. The air is warmed as it travels (as we will see later, cold air is an important asthma trigger). The windpipe, which is about 10–12cm long and about 2cm wide, is protected from crushing by rings of cartilage – rather like a vacuum cleaner hose.

The trachea then divides into two airways called the **major bronchi**, one for each lung. Rather like the branches of a tree, they divide some 10–25 times into thousands of smaller **bronchioles** –– each about 0.5mm in diameter – which end in the **alveoli**, little air sacs that look rather like cauliflower florets. This arrangement crams a vast surface area available for oxygen transfer into a relatively small space. The lungs contain some 300 million alveoli which, if spread out, would cover the surface of a tennis court.

Figure 1   The structure of the lungs

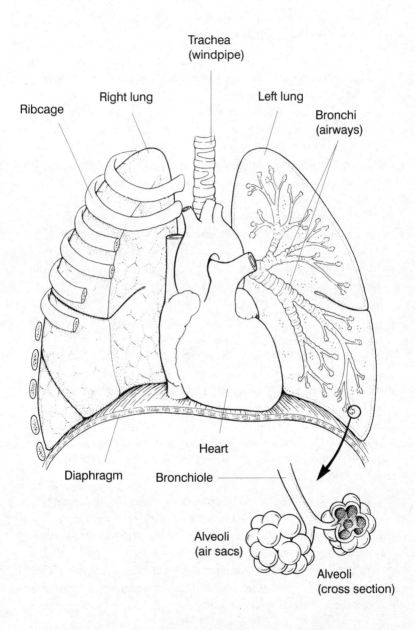

The exchange of gases

The alveoli are very thin and are covered by a network of tiny blood vessels, known as **capillaries**. It is here that oxygen is exchanged for waste carbon dioxide.

- Oxygen from air that has been breathed in dissolves in the fluid covering the alveoli, crosses the thin layer of cells, and is taken up by red blood cells.
- At the same time, the red blood cells release unwanted carbon dioxide, which moves across the alveoli into the air in the lung. This is expelled when you exhale.
- In the meantime, the oxygen-rich blood is carried from the lungs into the left side of the heart. From here the blood is pumped around the body.
- Once the red cells deliver their load of oxygen, they pick up a molecule of carbon dioxide and return to the right side of the heart.
- The next heartbeat brings the blood cells back to the lung and the whole process begins again.

Breathing

When you breathe in, your diaphragm contracts and flattens. At the same time, the intercostal muscles between the ribs shorten, pulling the ribcage up and out and increasing the space in the chest. This expansion pulls air into the lungs. The diaphragm and the intercostals then relax and the lungs return to their resting size. This expels the carbon-dioxide-rich air as you breathe out.

Respiration is controlled by an area of the brain known as the medulla, which acts like a thermostat.

- Receptors in the carotid artery – one of the blood vessels running up the neck – measure levels of oxygen and carbon dioxide in the blood. Nerves pass this information to the medulla, which lies at the base of the brain.
- When levels of carbon dioxide rise or levels of oxygen fall, the brain signals the diaphragm and intercostal muscles to increase or decrease the respiration rate.

This fine control allows respiration to adapt to the body's needs, so when you are asleep you need less oxygen than when you are running for a bus, and your respiration rate increases when you exercise. In contrast, when you rest your respiration rate slows.

The lungs' defence system

Each day 10,000 litres of air move in and out of the lungs. As well as oxygen, each breath carries particles, bacteria, viruses, fungi and pollutants deep inside the lungs. Not surprisingly, our lungs have evolved elaborate defences against the millions of potential invaders that permeate the air we inhale each day.

- The first line of defence is the hairs in the nostrils, which trap large particles. Further down the bronchi, particles become trapped in sticky mucus. The mucus is moved by tiny, hair-like protrusions (**cilia**) on cells lining the airways. The cilia waft the trapped particles up into the mouth and you swallow the mucus, which is then sterilised by enzymes and acid in your stomach. Severe uncontrolled asthma damages this 'mucociliary escalator', leaving you more vulnerable to infections.
- The second line of defence is the bronchioles. These are not rigid tubes but are flexible and surrounded by a ring of muscle. When this muscle contracts, it squeezes and narrows the airway in a reaction called **bronchoconstriction**. This prevents particles penetrating deep into the delicate alveoli. In asthma, it is the trigger that causes the bronchioles to narrow excessively in response to substances that leave most people unaffected.

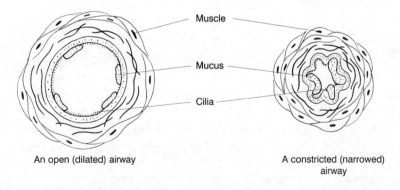

Muscle

Mucus

Cilia

An open (dilated) airway

A constricted (narrowed) airway

Figure 2 Open and narrowed airways

- White blood cells form the final line of defence. As well as oxygen your blood carries a number of white blood cells – so-called because they do not contain the red, oxygen-carrying pigment haemoglobin. White blood cells destroy invading micro-organisms. For example, **eosinophils** – a type of white blood cell that plays an important role in asthma – protect the body from parasitic infections.

Another type of white blood cell – the **T lymphocyte** – co-ordinates the body's immune response to ward off infection. For example, some T lymphocytes, made by the thymus glands at the base of the neck, stimulate the production of antibodies. Antibodies stick to the foreign invaders and act rather like a homing beacon for other white blood cells, by releasing a cocktail of chemicals – known as **inflammatory mediators** – that join the battle against viral, fungal or bacterial infections. In this way, antibodies encourage the white blood cells to destroy the invaders (for more detail see 'The immune response', below).

In asthma, however, the lungs' defensive process goes awry. The inflammatory mediators decribed above become biological terrorists fighting a civil war that eventually destroys the delicate fabric of the lung.

What goes wrong in asthma?

People with asthma seem to have over-sensitive immune systems that respond to **allergens** (substances that trigger an immune response) that most people find benign – so people with asthma may be hypersensitive to cat dander (shed skin and fur) or pollen. However, some react to non-allergic irritants, such as cold air. The inflammation that results when a sufferer comes into contact with an allergen leads to the symptoms of asthma: coughing, breathlessness and wheezing.

Until the mid-1970s, doctors believed that asthma was simply reversible bronchoconstriction (see above). We now know that bronchoconstriction arises from inflammation of the airways in the lung. Several pieces of evidence contributed to doctors' change of mind – which dramatically altered treatment. First, a technique known as bronchoscopy, developed during the 1960s, enabled doctors to take small samples of tissue from the lungs of people with asthma using a device that introduces a small camera inside the airways. This established that even people with mild asthma showed profound airway inflammation. Second, post-mortems of people who died suddenly from asthma revealed severe inflammation and plugs of mucus throughout their airways, though many of the patients had seemed to be relatively symptom-free until just before the attack. A combination of severe bronchoconstriction, thick mucus plugs and inflammation causing further narrowing of the airways seems to cause deaths from asthma – patients literally suffocate.

You may not be wheezy. You may not feel breathless. But the inflammation is there nonetheless, ready to flare when you encounter the right trigger. Understanding this inflammation and its triggers is the key to understanding asthma. The mechanism is complex – and this is probably the most difficult section of the book. But do not skip it. **Understanding the immune response that underlies asthma helps explain how the different drugs work, why certain tests help diagnose asthma and the importance of taking your drugs even when you feel well.**

The immune response

Inflammation is the body's response to injury. As we have seen, when the body encounters a virus, bacteria or fungus, white blood cells release a chemical cocktail of inflammatory mediators to combat the invader. Ironically, these chemicals also cause the symptoms of asthma. For example, one component of the chemical cocktail – histamine – can cause the muscles surrounding the airway to contract and lead to swelling of the lungs' lining. People with asthma seem to release these mediators in circumstances that would not affect most healthy people.

In other words, people with asthma appear to have an over-sensitive immune system that reacts to substances that most people find benign. So one person can walk through a field of grasses without harm, while if someone allergic to grass pollen took the same route they would develop the symptoms of hay fever or asthma. This over-sensitivity develops in two stages.

Sensitisation
The first time you encounter an allergic trigger (or allergen) your immune system is 'primed' to respond to future exposures. This process is known as sensitisation.

After the allergen penetrates deep into the lung and meets the delicate lining of the alveoli, one of the numerous white blood cells – the macrophages – breaks down the allergen. The body's natural defence system then works in two stages:

- **T lymphocytes** (page 18) recognise fragments of the allergen as a foreign invader. In response, they secrete a number of inflammatory mediators to carry messages between cells and co-ordinate the immune response. As a result, another type of lymphocyte – **B lymphocytes** derived from bone marrow – enters the fray.
- The inflammatory mediators released by T lymphocytes provoke some of the B lymphocytes into dividing and producing plasma cells. These plasma cells secrete an antibody called **immunoglobulin E (IgE)**.

IgE originally evolved to counter parasitic infections. The body fights bacterial infections with a different class of antibody. Following exposure to the allergen, IgE levels in the blood rise but, because plasma cells live for only a short time, drop after a few weeks. As this is the first time IgE has been produced, the first encounter does not give rise to symptoms. However, the immune system retains a long-living memory, programmed to react with much greater ferocity and mount an immune response next time you encounter the invader – a clear benefit if the invader is a bacterium – less so if it is pollen.

The next exposure
Antibodies protect your health. They attach to antigens (proteins on the surface of the cell) in order to render them harmless. During your next encounter with the allergen, the IgE antibody interacts with two types of white blood cells – **mast cells** in tissues and **basophils** in the blood.

- IgE is a Y-shaped protein: the long arm binds to the mast cell or basophil. Two adjacent IgE then bind a single antigen-presenting cell (the cell binds to one short arm on each IgE).
- This cross-linking stimulates the mast cell or basophil to release a cocktail of more than 20 inflammatory mediators from the granules inside the cell including histamine, leukotrienes, thromboxane, prostaglandins and platelet-activating factor. This is called degranulation.

As a result of these chemicals being released, you develop an acute asthma attack.

Figure 3   The allergic reaction in asthma

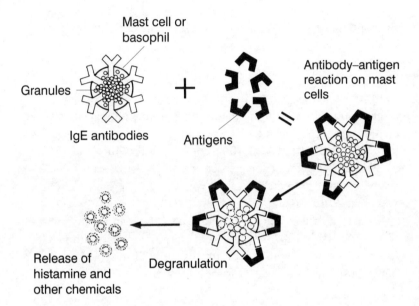

Adapted from a diagram in *Immunology Simplified* (OUP 1984)

What happens during an asthma attack?

Acute asthma attacks develop in two stages: an early phase that occurs within minutes of exposure to the allergen and a late phase that follows between six and eight hours later.

The early phase

Soon after exposure to the asthma trigger, blood vessels in the lung swell and become more leaky, or permeable. Fluid seeps from the blood into the surrounding tissues causing swelling (oedema). Furthermore, mucus secretion increases and the ring of muscle surrounding the bronchi contracts as bronchoconstriction (page 17) develops.

Bronchoconstriction evolved to keep allergens and other harmful chemicals out of the lung. However, in people with asthma the bronchoconstriction is excessive. It limits the amount of air flowing into the lung, causing wheezing and breathlessness. To make matters worse, the inflammatory mediators – chemicals released to combat the allergen – stimulate the nerves in the lung, triggering the coughing reflex and causing further bronchoconstriction.

The late phase
The swelling persists for several hours. In the meantime, two more types of white blood cells – neutrophils and eosinophils – migrate into the cells lining the bronchi. These white cells release chemical mediators that damage the delicate lining of the bronchioles (the epithelial layer). The chemicals also increase mucus secretion, trigger bronchoconstriction and leave the bronchi excessively sensitive or 'twitchy'. Often you may cough up mucus at the end of an asthma attack.

Eosinophil migration is a hallmark of asthma and is not typical of other allergic lung diseases. This late phase lasts about 8–12 hours following exposure to an allergen. However, bronchial hypersensitivity may persist for several days.

Long-term effects
Initially, the inflammation and symptoms characteristic of an asthma attack are reversible – either spontaneously or following treatment. However, prolonged inflammation irreparably damages the lung. The walls of the bronchioles become scarred and the delicate cilia are destroyed. Over time, the airway wall thickens and the number of mucus-secreting glands increases. When the asthma is well advanced, the ends of the bronchi become blocked with sticky mucus plugs. This process, known as remodelling, further reduces the airway diameter and makes a severe attack more likely – especially as the lungs are hypersensitive, and bronchoconstriction may be provoked following exposure to lower levels of the allergen. Patients may also react to non-allergic factors such as cold, heat and stress.

Can the effects be reversed?
The blockage of the airways that characterises asthma is made up of reversible and irreversible elements:

- Hyper-responsiveness, oedema and bronchoconstriction are more or less reversible – bronchodilators (see **Chapter 5**) can reverse bronchoconstriction within minutes.
- A mucus plug may take six weeks or longer to be relieved.
- In severe cases, airway remodelling and scarring are irreversible.

It is therefore vital to diagnose and treat asthma before it becomes irreversible. So what symptoms should you watch for?

The symptoms of asthma

The inflammation that causes asthma means that the airways narrow easily in response to a wide range of triggers and you may develop a number of symptoms. However, you may not experience all of these:

- shortness of breath
- wheezing
- chest tightness
- coughing up phlegm or feeling congested
- coughing (in children and in early or mild asthma, cough may be the main or only symptom).

During an acute asthma attack, you may develop a number of other symptoms:

- breaths in may seem 'snatched' and breaths out prolonged
- rapid breathing (hyperventilation)
- increased heart rate – an asthma attack can be terrifying
- a feeling of suffocation.

The combination of profound bronchoconstriction and increased mucus production can completely block the airways. As a result, airflow stops and in some severe cases the patient may suffocate (known as 'status asthmaticus').

What makes asthma different?
There are some important points to note about asthma that distinguish it from other respiratory diseases.

- The obstruction in asthma is reversible – unlike that in chronic bronchitis, emphysema and cystic fibrosis.

- Bronchoconstriction and mucus plugs occur throughout the bronchial tree.
- Lung function approaches normal levels between attacks, unlike chronic airway obstruction.
- Inflammation and hyper-reactivity occur even if you feel well. As a result, almost all asthma sufferers need to take medicine to control the underlying inflammation to reduce the number and severity of their attacks, even when they are symptom-free.
- Symptoms are intermittent – for example, about half of all children with asthma show a seasonal variation in symptoms (reflecting allergens in the environment, colds or viral infections).

Types of asthma

Mild, moderate and severe asthma

The severity of asthma symptoms in different people varies widely. Some people experience only occasional, mild symptoms. Others endure severe, debilitating attacks on encountering a specific allergen (e.g. cat dander). A number of people live with chronic, incapacitating asthma on a daily basis – indeed, one in ten people with asthma have severely compromised lifestyles. Doctors usually describe asthma as being mild, moderate and severe according to the following criteria:

- **Mild asthma** – symptoms that do not interfere with sleep or daily activities; or bouts of coughing and wheezing that occur less than once a month.
- **Moderate asthma** – attacks that occur no more than once a week.
- **Severe asthma** – recurrent, troublesome attacks during most days or nights. Severe asthma may need treatment with regular courses of oral steroids (**Chapter 5**).

Asthma may be chronic (long-lasting) or acute (occurring in isolated attacks, known as **exacerbations**). So you could have chronic mild asthma or acute severe asthma, or you could experience daily symptoms punctuated by acute exacerbations. In other words, asthma ranges from mild, intermittent disease (e.g. following exercise) to a chronic, severe condition where patients endure daily, almost continual, breathlessness.

While severe symptoms tend to be caused by more intense inflammation, the frequency and severity of asthma attacks may not directly reflect the underlying inflammation. Indeed, some patients feel fine until they suffer a severe attack. These patients often think that their asthma worsened rapidly, but careful questioning usually reveals that their condition deteriorated slowly over a few weeks. **Brittle asthma** describes the condition of a patient whose asthma genuinely worsens suddenly and inexplicably.

This poor ability on the part of people with asthma to gauge the severity of their symptoms means that they should monitor their lung function regularly. This is done using a device called a peak flow meter, which can act as an early warning system of an imminent asthma attack. **Chapter 4** has more on peak flow meters.

Cough-variant asthma

Coughing is an important asthma symptom. It is however often trivialised, under-diagnosed and under-treated.

We frequently find a cough irritating, yet it is a reflex designed to protect our lungs. A cough expels foreign particles and excess mucus from the respiratory tract. As a result, it can be a symptom of many respiratory diseases. Chronic cough is common – up to 23 per cent of non-smokers suffer from a cough that lasts more than three weeks at some point during their lives. However, in nine out of ten patients doctors may be able to identify a cause – often asthma.

About 80 per cent of people with asthma endure daily bouts of coughing. Some asthma patients experience a dry, non-productive cough. Others produce copious amounts of clear or yellow sputum. The yellow colour arises from the large number of eosinophils that have invaded the lung during the late phase of an attack (page 22).

Nocturnal asthma

Between two-thirds and three-quarters of people with asthma find that their wheezing and other asthma symptoms are worse at night and early in the morning – a condition known as nocturnal asthma. Furthermore, fatal asthma attacks are more likely to occur at night than during the day. Figures show that 11–39 per cent of people with asthma wake with asthma every night; 16–24 per cent wake 3–6 nights a week; and 25–53 per cent wake one night a month.

Nocturnal asthma leaves patients sleepy, irritable and tired during the day. This obviously increases the risk of accidents and causes considerable stress. Moreover, a recent survey suggested that people with asthma were twice as likely to report sleeping difficulties and early morning waking as the general population. But people with asthma should steer clear of sleeping pills (hypnotics). If sedated, you are less able to notice – and therefore treat – a nocturnal asthma attack.

What causes nocturnal asthma?

All diseases are felt more intensely in the still of the night. However, there are biological reasons why asthma tends to deteriorate in the small hours. The diameter of the bronchioles does not remain constant throughout the day. Instead, they are at their narrowest at around 3–4a.m. and widest between midday and 4p.m. This pattern, known as diurnal variation, affects everyone – even people without asthma.

Natural reduction of airway calibre due to diurnal variation can be intensified if the sufferer is experiencing the late phase of an asthma attack (page 22). Other factors include airway cooling as the external temperature drops – cold air has a detrimental effect on the airways – and whether or not your immune system is more active at night. However, many patients experience their worst chest tightness, lung function and wheezing in the morning when they attempt to get up, due to the combination of narrow bronchi and increased physical activity. Doctors call this the 'morning dip'.

Take action on nocturnal asthma

Nocturnal asthma is a warning signal that your asthma is poorly controlled. People suffering from nocturnal asthma are more likely to have severe asthma and poor lung function. Yet despite nocturnal asthma being a common, treatable phenomenon, many people regard it as a burden they have to live with – even though it may undermine their quality of life. Up to half do not inform their doctors about nocturnal symptoms. In one survey, 41 per cent of people with asthma felt that night-time symptoms had to be accepted, while 37 per cent felt nocturnal asthma was nothing to worry about. Ironically, modern drugs are available which can alleviate nocturnal asthma.

So do not ignore nocturnal asthma. It may herald a worsening control of symptoms – and underscore the need for reviewing your treatment. If you are experiencing the symptoms of nocturnal asthma, make an appointment to see your GP.

CHAPTER 2

THE ASTHMA TRIGGERS

IN most sufferers, asthma is an allergic or atopic (the Greek for 'alien') disease – the immune system over-reacts when the body's defence systems are breached by an foreign invader known as an allergen, as described in **Chapter 1**. However, most people with asthma tend to be sensitive to a number of triggers. For example, you may react to cigarette smoke, pollen and stress at different times.

A few asthma sufferers appear to be exceptions to this rule. In the condition known as **non-allergic asthma**, patients display typical symptoms of asthma but the disease does not appear to be provoked by any allergen in particular. However, just because doctors cannot identify the allergen it does not mean that the patient's asthma does not have an allergic foundation. The likelihood of suffering from non-allergic asthma increases as you get older (page 176) – this may reflect hypersensitivity following years of uncontrolled inflammation in the lung, or be due to other respiratory conditions. So the airways may narrow in response to a range of triggers – cold air, tobacco smoke, pollution, dust, perfumes, cleaning agents and so on. In these cases, uncovering the primary cause is almost impossible.

Isolating the culprits

The identification of your asthma triggers can be a vital step towards improved management of your condition. Once you know what allergen is causing your asthma symptoms, efforts can be made to avoid the trigger(s) in question and you can exercise self-management measures to help yourself cope. This may prove impossible, especially if the trigger is a common one: e.g. pollen, the house dust mite or dander (shed skin and fur) from a loved pet. Nevertheless, there are certain steps you can take to minimise your exposure to triggers (see **Chapter 8**).

Some triggers are simple to identify – a child who wheezes only after running may have exercise-induced asthma. Others are harder to identify, although doctors can use a number of tests to pin down the suspect (see pages 71–83).

Animal and insect triggers

House dust mites

It is an unpleasant thought, but your bed and carpets are infested with millions of tiny creatures that feed on your dead skin. These house dust mites are the commonest allergen among people with asthma: 60–80 per cent of people with asthma (and 20 per cent of the general population) are sensitive to the house dust mite.

The mites live in warm, humid conditions – ideal breeding grounds are bedding, upholstery, carpets, air-conditioning systems, children's soft toys, clothing, footwear, and even, according to one study, the scalp. People tend to be allergic to either the faeces of the mite, its outer layer (which is shed) or enzymes in the mites' saliva.

These invisible squatters are present in incredible numbers. Studies from the Netherlands suggest that up to 555 mites are found in every gram of dust from upholstery, 450 mites in every gram of dust from mattresses and 280 mites in every gram of dust from carpets. However, other studies suggest that there can be as many as 5,000 mites per gram of dust. To put these alarming-sounding figures into context:

- 100 mites per gram of dust in a mattress will not increase the risk of developing asthma
- 110–1,000 mites increase the risk of developing asthma five-fold
- over 1,000 mites increase the risk of developing asthma eight-fold (a risk similar to that of developing lung cancer among smokers).

Cockroaches

Cockroaches are another common, if underestimated, allergen, especially in deprived inner city areas. In America, up to 58 per cent of people with allergic asthma are sensitive to the cockroach. In Europe the figure appears to be lower – proportions range from 6.3 per cent in Switzerland to 25.7 per cent in Spain. Nevertheless, if you are being tested for sensitivity to various allergens through skin prick testing (see page 78), you might want to suggest including cockroaches as a potential trigger, especially if you live in the inner city.

Pets

After the house dust mite, pets are the commonest cause of domestic allergy. Certain pets trigger asthma and other allergic lung diseases. For example, some pet owners develop allergies to cat or dog dander or those animals' hair, saliva and urine.

- About 50 per cent of people with asthma are sensitive to aller-gens produced by either cats, dogs, or both.
- People who own pigeons, budgerigars or other birds may become allergic to their feathers – a problem known as pigeon-fancier's lung.
- Symptoms caused by pets tend to worsen during the winter, when the house tends to be less well ventilated and you remain indoors more.

Pet allergens can become extremely widespread throughout the house. For example, the cat allergen, which is present in small air-borne particles, can pervade dust on the floor, soft furnishings and the wall. It tends to be very difficult to remove, evading the most stringent cleaning, and is likely to remain in the home for several months even if the offending cat is removed.

Emotion

Strong emotions – anger, stress or joy – can trigger asthma. Some children with asthma cough when they laugh hard or become excited, for example. Older children and adults often find that their asthma gets worse at times of stress – e.g. during an argument, while taking exams or when they get married. Moreover, asthma can exert a heavy psychological toll on people who have the condition, which may further undermine how well they control their symptoms (see **Chapter 3**).

While nerves and stress do *not* cause asthma, they can exacerbate the underlying tendency. It is therefore important to bolster your defences against stress – **Chapter 9** offers some suggestions on complementary therapies that not only reduce stress but may also directly improve asthma.

Exercise-induced asthma

Exercise is good for you, but it is also a common asthma trigger. A combination of exercise, hyperventilation (panting) and cold air causes bronchoconstriction in about three-quarters of people with asthma – although for some exercise is the main, or only, trigger. These people suffer from 'exercise-induced asthma'.

What happens in exercise-induced asthma?

Almost 2,000 years ago, physicians noted that physical exercise could provoke airway obstruction; it has taken that length of time even to begin to understand why.

- When you participate in a physical activity, your heart rate rises and your muscles demand more oxygen. Initially, the bronchi dilate (widen) to allow more air into your lungs in response to your muscles' request.
- In people with exercise-induced asthma the bronchi then constrict, reaching their narrowest after 5–8 minutes of intense exercise. This bronchoconstriction can cause feelings of chest pain and the patient may cough and wheeze.
- Oddly, the asthma may improve on continuing the exercise. This is because exercise produces a natural hormone, adrenaline, which acts in the same way as a bronchodilator (**Chapter 5**) – as levels of adrenaline rise in the blood, symptoms are relieved.
- Most people recover within 20–60 minutes, although a few develop a late reaction 3–13 hours later.

What factors contribute to exercise-induced asthma?

Several factors may play a role in exercise-induced asthma, including the climate, the patient's underlying airway hypersensitivity and the intensity of the exercise.

Cold, dry air is far more likely to provoke an asthma attack than warm, humid air. This may be one reason why many people with asthma find that the weather affects their symptoms, though why this happens is less clear. Some researchers believe that cold, dry air increases water loss from the lungs. All animals narrow their bronchi to prevent the lungs from drying out; as a result, the airway muscles contract. But among people with exercise-induced asthma, the narrowing of the airways is excessive. This triggers the symptoms of asthma (see **Chapter 1**). Another theory holds that a fall in airway temperature leads to swelling and congestion in susceptible people. Others believe the airways may narrow as a result of the cooling followed by rapid re-warming that occurs as the patient breathes in and out.

While the cause of exercise-induced asthma remains something of a mystery, it is clear that some exercises are more likely to provoke asthma than others.

- running tends to trigger asthma more frequently than indoor exercises
- winter sports – skiing and ice skating – are difficult for many people with asthma
- cycling, cross-country skiing and basketball are more likely to cause an attack
- swimming and gymnastics are less likely to provoke symptoms.

Diagnosing exercise-induced asthma

Diagnosing exercise-induced asthma presents a problem. Doctors measuring the lung function of an exercising patient usually regard a 15 per cent reduction in the 'forced expiratory volume', (page 76) – a measure of lung function – as signifying exercise-induced asthma. But should athletes be judged by the same criteria, where success is measured in fractions of a second? Moreover, breathlessness and chest pain, though symptomatic of asthma, can also be a sign of heart disease – or simply being unfit. As a result, exercise-induced asthma may go unrecognised and untreated. So what should you watch for?

- Children with exercise-induced asthma tend to cough, wheeze and complain of chest pains soon after starting exercise. The symptoms get worse for a few minutes and last for about half an hour.
- Often the first sign among older children and adults is a 'locker room cough' following activity, or feeling 'out of shape'.

Ironically, exercise-induced asthma is easily treated. For tips on how to reduce your risk of developing the condition, see page 172.

Exercise-induced asthma in elite athletes

The symptoms of exercise-induced asthma are found even among elite athletes. A study of American athletes during the 1984 Summer Olympics found that 11 per cent of the team suffered from exercise-induced asthma, though only 26 per cent of this group reported a history of asthma. The remainder coughed, wheezed or felt their chest was tight after strenuous exercise (see table). Cyclists and runners were discovered to be the most likely to develop exercise-induced asthma. However, a tendency to exercise-induced asthma need not compromise performance. The 67 people with exercise-induced asthma won 41 medals – 15 of which were gold.

Table 1: Symptoms of exercise-induced asthma among elite athletes

Symptom	Per cent showing symptom
Cough	50
Chest congestion	40
Chest tightness	36
Wheeze	25

Food allergies

Claiming that foods trigger your asthma is almost fashionable. While food allergies are a real, and serious, clinical problem, the role of food in triggering asthma is often overstated. One study interviewed almost 19,000 people. Of these, about a fifth declared themselves to be 'intolerant' to certain foods – usually chocolate, additives, citrus fruits and shellfish. However, only 1.4–1.8 per cent proved to be truly intolerant when their susceptibilities were scientifically assessed (see 'Dietary challenge tests', page 81).

Allergic or intolerant?

One problem is that many people confuse food allergies and food intolerance.

- **Food allergies** involve the immune system, which triggers a reaction and produces specific immunoglobulin E (IgE) – the allergy antibody – when the sufferer comes into contact with the culprit food. People with food intolerance do not produce specific IgE.
- **Food intolerance** – though responsible for some unpleasant symptoms that may mimic those of an allergic reaction – results from a number of non-allergic causes, such as the subject lacking an enzyme that digests food; or a substance in the food that irritates the gut lining or contains a chemical that triggers asthma.

The following example illustrates how closely food intolerance can mimic food allergy. Some foods contain histamine, a chemical responsible for some symptoms of asthma, as seen in **Chapter 1** (page 20). The histamine in red wine can trigger sneezing, flushing, headache, itching and breathlessness in sensitive (though not allergic) people – sometimes after as little as a single glass. In one study of 22 people intolerant of red wine, two developed mild asthma attacks and showed a 30 per cent reduction in lung function after drinking the wine.

Cheese, fish, sausages, certain vegetables and beer also contain histamine – although levels are highest in wine. This is one good reason to limit the amount of alcohol you drink.

How sensitive is sensitive?

A hypersensitivity to peanuts is probably the best-known true allergy. Peanuts are not nuts but a legume related to peas and beans. However, in susceptible people a wide range of foods including chestnuts, bananas and avocados can trigger hypersensitivity that can develop into symptoms similar to asthma. Indeed, sometimes you do not even have to eat the food to develop a reaction. Furthermore, many patients are **cross-sensitive**. So patients allergic to kiwi fruit tend to show strong reactions to apple and hazelnut and weaker reactions to carrot, potato and avocado, though no one knows what underlies this odd relationship. Many people who are allergic to fruit also react to latex – a leading cause of occupational allergies, including asthma (see 'Occupational triggers', page 43).

Some people are exquisitely sensitive to certain foods – just handling certain foods is enough to provoke an asthma attack. For example, some people are allergic to raw potatoes – even peeling the spuds triggers rhinitis (hay fever) and asthma attacks. In one case, a housewife developed asthma after boiling Swiss chard (a vegetable). Other people have suffered asthma attacks after peeling green beans and handling raw rice.

People with a confirmed food allergy should check the label of food products carefully to avoid any unpleasant encounters. It is, however, important to keep the risks of food allergies in perspective.

Doctors tested 100 patients suffering from hay fever for sensitivity to avocado using skin prick tests (page 78):

- 21 people tested positive
- 8 per cent reported developing symptoms – such as an itchy mouth and throat and a swollen tongue – after eating avocados
- 8 per cent developed asthma symptoms such as wheeziness and chest tightness
- 7 per cent showed raised levels of IgE – the allergy antibody.

Another study assessed 1,126 four-year-olds. Of these:

- 22 per cent developed asthma or wheezing
- 25 per cent had eczema
- 17 per cent had recurrent blocked noses – which may imply hay fever.

The children then underwent a skin prick test to test their sensitivity to various allergens. The table shows that food allergies lag well behind house dust mites and moulds.

Table 2: The percentage of four-year-old children sensitive to allergens

Allergen	Per cent sensitive
House dust mite	12.2
Grass	7.7
Cats	5.6
Alternaria (outdoor mould)	4.9
Dogs	2.3
Cladosporium (outdoor mould)	1.8
Milk	1.5
Peanuts	1.1
Egg	0.9
Wheat	0.3
Soya	0.1

These findings illustrate two important points. First, food allergies are rare even among people with confirmed allergies. Secondly, just because you are sensitive to a food on skin prick testing does not necessarily mean that it triggers your asthma, as will be explained in **Chapter 4**. Indeed, taking food allergies too seriously may mean you exclude certain foods from your diet and run the risk of nutritional deficiencies.

The role of additives and preservatives

In a few people – perhaps 3–15 people in every 1,000 of the population – asthma is triggered by additives and preservatives. Overall, just two per cent of children with allergic diseases are sensitive to additives and preservatives. However, some people with asthma are more sensitive to metabisulphite, a preservative used in dried fruits, pickles, sausages, fruit and on certain vegetables. In these people, metabisulphite can trigger an asthma attack, possibly because the gas sulphur dioxide is released during cooking (the pollutant irritates the lungs). In addition, people with aspirin-induced asthma (see opposite) may cross-react to the dye tartrazine (E102), which is used to colour foods and some medicines yellow or orange.

The table below shows some common food colours and preservatives that may be linked to asthma. Check the packet carefully to avoid these potential triggers.

Table 3: Food colours and preservatives linked to asthma

E number	Name
102	Tartrazine
104	Quinoline yellow
110	Sunset yellow
210	Benzoic acid
211	Sodium benzoate
212	Potassium benzoate
213	Calcium benzoate
214–219	Hydroxy benzoate salts
220–227	Sodium metabisulphite

Foods containing salicylates

A group of related chemicals, known as salicylates, can trigger asthma in sensitive people. They include aspirin (see 'Aspirin-induced asthma', below), but are also used as food preservatives and occur naturally in certain foods – see the table below for a list of foods that may contain salicylates. Total avoidance of these foods is impracticable, but watch out for and steer clear of those foods that seem to particularly affect you.

SOME FOODS THAT MAY CONTAIN SALICYLATES

Some alcoholic drinks
Some breads
Some breakfast cereals
Cake mix
Chewing gum
Chocolate
Cooked meats
Fruit (apples, apricots, cherries, grapes, oranges, peaches, plums, raisins, raspberries, strawberies)

Hot dogs
Ice-cream
Liquorice
Margarine
Pasteurised cheese
Sandwich spreads
Some soft drinks
Toothpaste
Vegetables (except pickles, tomato and cucumber)

Aspirin-induced asthma

Aspirin sensitivity is fairly common among people with asthma. Doctors can diagnose aspirin-induced asthma by performing certain tests (see pages 80–81).

- Estimates vary, but depending on the way in which asthma is defined, 2–28 per cent of people with asthma wheeze after taking aspirin *or* a related class of drugs known as **non-steroidal anti-inflammatory drugs (NSAIDs)**, widely used to treat inflammatory diseases such as arthritis, sports injuries and headaches.
- Middle-aged women are at especially high risk – some three women are affected for every two men.
- In some cases, just 30mg of aspirin – about a tenth of a normal aspirin dose – is enough to trigger an attack that includes severe bronchoconstriction, runny nose, flushing, itching and a rash. The symptoms usually develop within a few minutes.
- Most people with aspirin-induced asthma also suffer from chronic hay fever and sinusitis, and may develop growths inside the nose called polyps.
- Aspirin sensitivity may be a marker of disease severity. In one study, almost a quarter of asthma sufferers admitted to hospital with a life-threatening attack were aspirin-sensitive. In another, 40 per cent of people with asthma dependent on steroids to control their symptoms were found to be sensitive to aspirin, compared to 19 per cent of those who did not need steroids.

What causes aspirin sensitivity?

Why some people with asthma become sensitive to aspirin is not fully understood. The sensitivity is probably not caused by an immune reaction. Some doctors believe that NSAIDs (see above) throw the balance of inflammatory mediators into disarray. Aspirin and other NSAIDs act by blocking the production of prostaglandins – hormone-like compounds that are important mediators of both pain and inflammation. NSAIDs may therefore relieve the ache and swelling that underlie arthritis or other, similar conditions. However, in some people this action stimulates the production of mediators – including leukotrienes (page 20 – that lead to bronchoconstriction.

Fortunately, aspirin-induced asthma can be treated. Where possible, sufferers should avoid aspirin – if you require aspirin for a serious condition, e.g. to thin your blood following a heart attack, you should contact your GP. To avoid the risk of drugs triggering aspirin-induced symptoms, make sure that your doctor or pharmacist knows you suffer from asthma. You will probably be advised to avoid using aspirin and ibuprofen – both available over-the-counter – or similar NSAIDs, as either tablets or creams. You should also take care to avoid certain foods that contain salicylates (see box above).

Nasal congestion may respond to decongestants (though these are not recommended long-term), anti-histamines or nasal steroids. Polyps inside the nose can be removed by a surgeon. Desensitisation (page 133) may be particularly effective for aspirin-sensitive asthma, with 31 per cent of patients reporting improvements in their asthma and 68 per cent describing less nasal congestion.

Pollution

Whether poor air quality causes asthma is controversial. There is little doubt, however, that pollution exacerbates asthma and other respiratory diseases. The London Smog of 1952 – when a mixture of fog, smoke and chemical fumes hung so thickly in the air that people could barely see a few yards in front of them – claimed 4,000 lives in excess of the norm, mostly from respiratory illnesses. The public outcry led to the 1956 Clean Air Act, which made anything but smokeless fuel illegal in central zones.

But at least you could see smog. Today's pollutants tend to be almost invisible. If you get the chance, look over a major city from a hill on a summer's day. You will see a haze – this is visible evidence of pollution. When you wash your hair after walking around in a city for a day, the shampoo sometimes runs dark when you rinse your hair for the same reason. And statistics show that levels of traffic pollution could be getting worse: in 1989, British people owned 23 million motor vehicles. By 2025, the number is expected to rise to 50 million.

The link with asthma

Parents often blame pollution for the rise in childhood asthma – although there is little hard evidence to support this. In fact, some experts believe indoor air quality is more important. But it is clear that pollution exacerbates asthma and may make the difference between having a predisposition to asthma and developing symptoms, or between having mild, intermittent symptoms and developing chronic moderate symptoms.

Furthermore, asthma tends to be more common in the cities of developing countries than in the rural areas.

- Japanese studies show that people living near busy roads are more likely to become sensitive to cedar tree pollen than those living in a less polluted environment. Pollen counts are similar in both areas.

- A study from Munich in Germany examined lung function and breathlessness among children aged 9–11 years. The greater the number of cars in the area, the worse the overall lung function and the more children tended to become breathless. Chronic bronchitis and allergic diseases tend to be more common in the polluted cities of the former East Germany.

- A Swedish study compared children growing up two towns. In the first, children were exposed to sulphur dioxide and fluoride pollution pumped from an aluminium smelter and emissions from other heavy industries. The other town had no polluting industry. Results indicated that children exposed to sulphur dioxide during the first year of life and fluoride during the first three years were more likely to develop bronchial hyper-responsiveness when aged 7–13. Reports from Germany corroborate these findings.

So there is a growing body of circumstantial evidence to suggest that poor air quality exacerbates asthma. Indeed, a Department of Health report suggests that pollution exacerbates symptoms in about five per cent of people with asthma (while maintaining that pollution does not cause the disease).

Yet pollution is a complex chemical cocktail, the effects of which are difficult to disentangle. It can contain some, or all, of the following.

- **'Acid air'** is produced through a chemical reaction between light, nitrogen dioxide and sulphur dioxide. The reaction forms tiny clouds containing drops of sulphuric and nitric acid. Eventually, this leads to acid rain. If you have seen pictures of the devastation wrought by acid rain on forests, imagine what it can do to your lungs.

- **Carbon monoxide**, mainly emitted from cars, binds to haemoglobin, thereby interfering with red blood cells' ability to carry oxygen from the lungs to other organs. People suffering from heart disease are especially vulnerable to carbon monoxide's effects and the gas may inhibit foetal growth and mental development. However, cigarette smoke is a far more important source of carbon monoxide than cars.

- **Nitrogen dioxide** – another gas produced by cars and power stations – irritates the lining of the lung. Found at high levels by the sides of busy roads, nitrogen dioxide can make breathing difficult for people with asthma. Indeed, severe nitrogen dioxide pollution during December 1991 may be linked to a small increase in mortality. In the home, gas cooking or heating increases levels of nitrogen dioxide. Nitrogen dioxide levels above 100 parts per billion of air indicate poor air quality.

- **Ozone** is produced from the chemical reaction that occurs when light falls on nitrogen dioxide and hydrocarbons – so ozone levels tend to be highest on bright, warm summer days. Related to oxygen, ozone is a highly reactive gas that irritates the nose, lungs, eyes and throat. Ozone levels above 90 parts per billion can trigger breathing problems, including asthma, among vulnerable people and those taking strenuous exercise.

- **Smoke** produced by traffic, power stations and coal fires consists of a range of particles. Larger particles are trapped in the upper airways and nose. However, particles below 10μm in diameter – you could fit 100 of these in a centimetre – and particularly those below 2.5μm seem to pose a specific health hazard. Known as 'particulate pollution', these smaller particles travel deep into the lung where they irritate the delicate lining. Furthermore, smaller particles are often rich in a group of chemicals known as polyaromatic hydrocarbons, which may cause cancer. Diesel engines tend to emit more smoke than petrol engines and particles from diesel fumes may stick to the surface of the pollen, making it more likely to trigger an asthma attack.

- **Sulphur dioxide**, a gas produced by power stations, diesel engines and coal fires, was the main culprit during the smogs. Sulphur dioxide constricts the airways, making breathing difficult, especially in young children. Overall, the Clean Air Act (see page 39) means that sulphur dioxide levels have fallen, although levels remain high in some industrial areas.

So, pollution exacerbates asthma symptoms. On the one hand, some doctors believe the link is stronger than that admitted by the Department of Health (above). However, others believe that the current emphasis on pollution as a cause for asthma provides a con- venient excuse for people who do not want to believe that it is their smoking or the home environment that is causing the symptoms.

Until the extent of pollution's involvement in asthma is unrav- elled, it seems prudent to take precautions. Avoid going out when the air quality is poor and do not exercise outdoors on polluted days (remember that this also applies to exercising in front of an open window). You may also want to increase your dose of anti- inflammatory drug (see **Chapter 5**) during high-pollution days – discuss this with your doctor.

Pollen and spores

In 1981, doctors in Barcelona were baffled. They faced a dramatic rise in the number of adults being admitted to hospital suffering from asthma – but only at certain times. After two years of careful detective work, the physicians traced the source – airborne dust from the loading and unloading of soya bean at the city's harbour.

Plants and moulds are common asthma triggers. They repro- duce by spreading tiny specks of pollen and minute spores that float on the wind, so you are liable to breathe them in – and it is the pollens and spores, rather than the plants and moulds them- selves, that usually trigger symptoms.

The plants and fungi responsible for inciting asthma attacks vary during the year.

- **Trees** pollinate between March and May.
- **Grasses** pollinate between May and early July.
- **Outdoor moulds** such as *Alternaria* and *Cladosporium* release spores in the early spring, but the largest increase occurs dur- ing the late summer and autumn.
- **Pollen** levels fluctuate throughout the day, tending to peak in the early morning and late afternoon. In the countryside, the evening pollen peaks occur earlier than in the city. In the city

the evening peaks tend to be greater than the morning peaks.

- If you are allergic to pollen, listen out for the pollen counts on the television and radio. You can also contact the National Asthma Campaign★ pollen line during summer.

Air turbulence and sudden damp conditions trigger the release of fungal spores. Climatic changes also seem to be altering the distri bution of certain pollens and spores. For example, growing seasons are beginning earlier in warmer climates so birch and alder pollen appear to be released earlier now than in previous years. Moreover, farming is changing – an increased number of hectares are being switched from grasses, cereals and sugar beet to sunflowers and rape seed for their oil; or are being given over to forestry and housing development. This is good news if you are allergic to grass pollen, but not if your asthma is triggered by rape pollen.

Occupational triggers

Occupational asthma was first noted among grain workers in the eighteenth century. The number of people affected by allergic disease increased during the Industrial Revolution, and now recent American studies suggest that occupational triggers cause up to 15 per cent of asthma cases. In the UK, the figure may be less – perhaps two per cent of all asthma cases are attributed to occupational triggers.

- Some 500 people a year are diagnosed as suffering from occupational asthma; doctors suspect that the true figure may be three times this.
- Each year 1,000–2,000 people are forced to give up work because of occupational asthma. Some do not find alternative jobs.
- One study surveyed 34 people who developed occupational asthma. Of these, 20 either lost or changed their job as a result of their asthma and 25 felt they suffered financially.
- In another survey, 49 out of 79 people with occupational asthma were either unemployed or on lower wages than they would have otherwise expected.

Perhaps as a result of the economic toll, one in ten people with occupational asthma does not change their job – placing their work over their health. Industrial injuries payments were not widely available before 1990 for occupational asthma and, in any case, do not offset the lost earnings. Occupational asthma is clearly a major economic and social problem.

What triggers occupational asthma?

Over 200 materials found in the workplace are linked to occupational asthma, including flour and grain, latex, platinum salts, isocyanates and wood dust. These are known as sensitisers. In addition, gases, fumes, vapour and airborne particles can all trigger asthma.

Occupational asthma triggers can be divided into two main groups:

- The commonest type emerges after a latent period, during which time the sufferer's allergic response becomes established – e.g. the number of workers sensitive to flour increases from about 10 per cent of apprentice bakers to maybe 30 per cent of experienced bakers.
- More rarely, some irritants can immediately trigger an attack without a latent period. In isolated instances, such as the soya bean asthma epidemic in Barcelona (see page 42) and in the case of certain insecticides, sensitisers directly trigger bronchoconstriction.

The number of people affected differs between industries. For example, bakers, grain handlers, farm workers feeding animals and other people working with flours are at increased risk of developing occupational asthma – and not only from the flour itself.

- Isocynanates – chemicals used in the manufacture of plastics, foams and adhesives – are the commonest cause of occupational asthma, accounting for a fifth of all reported cases.
- Enzymes are increasingly used in the food, chemical and drug industries. They are proteins and can trigger an immune reaction. As a result, people working with enzymes are at risk of developing allergies and asthma.
- Natural rubber (latex) is another notorious asthma trigger – especially among health care workers, for instance – e.g. one in

20 people involved in the manufacture of latex gloves and one in 40 people working in hospitals suffer from asthma induced by latex.

- Storage mites, fungi, insects and flour additives can all trigger asthma. In addition to wheat, buckwheat, chickpea and soya bean flours can all provoke symptoms.
- Dyes, wood dusts and foods including garlic and asparagus have been linked to occupational asthma (see 'Food allergies', page 33). Flowers and some seeds may also trigger asthma.

Provided occupational asthma is treated promptly and the patient is not exposed again to the irritant, most people recover. Be on the alert for the warning signs listed on page 170, and if you think you are beginning to suffer from occupational asthma it is important to consult your doctor – in the interests of both your physical and financial health. See also pages 170–2.

Smoking

Despite the dangers, many people with asthma smoke. Adolescents may smoke to relieve the stress of growing up with asthma, or because of peer pressure. Adults with asthma may also smoke to relieve stress, or to give themselves a mental boost.

All smokers put their lives at risk, but smoking is particularly harmful for people with asthma – smokers tend to have more severe asthma than non-smokers. And it is not only your own health that you are damaging. Millions of people continue to put their children's health at risk from passive smoking, despite there being no doubt that passive smoking impairs lung function. A study of almost 11,000 Greek children aged 9–12 found that children brought up in homes where the parents smoked more than five cigarettes a day were more than twice as likely to cough, produce sputum and wheeze – three hallmarks of asthma – than those living in non-smoking households.

Maternal smoking is especially dangerous – mothers still tend to spend more time with their children than fathers. A Dutch study of 1,800 primary school children found that those whose mothers smoked more than ten cigarettes a day were more likely to develop chronic cough, shortness of breath and wheeziness. Lung function was also impaired. Paternal smoking had no effect. Despite the apparently negligible effect of fathers' habits, there is probably no safe level for passive smoking. Doctors from Rome studied the effect of environmental tobacco smoke in public places on 300 10- to 15-year-olds. They found that even occasional exposure lowered lung function. Overall, passive smoking at least doubles the risk that the child will contract lung infections.

The message is clear: don't let your children breathe someone else's smoke. Eliminating passive smoking could go a long way to reducing the risk of children developing asthma. **Chapter 8** offers advice on how to quit.

Viral infections

Viral infections are another common asthma trigger. Many children find their asthma deteriorates when they catch a cold, for instance. Indeed, cold viruses can be isolated from 80–85 per cent of children who suffer an asthma attack. Viruses may also account for about a third of adult cases, leading to a fall in lung function as well as triggering cough and wheeze. To make matters worse, people with asthma may be six times more likely to develop a respiratory tract infection than those without asthma, possibly because scarring due to both asthma and the infection damages the mucociliary escalator (page 17). Mucus, which is produced continuously, is an ideal breeding-ground for bacteria and viruses, so ensure that you are vaccinated against influenza (page 194).

Apart from triggering an exacerbation, some infections – such as respiratory syncytial virus (RSV) – seem to predispose to asthma. For example, one study compared children who developed bronchiolitis – a lung infection mainly caused by RSV – with those who contracted pneumonia before the age of two and a group of children who did not develop either disease. The children were then re-examined 7–8 years later. Fifteen per cent of the children suffering from bronchiolitis developed asthma, compared with seven per cent who contracted pneumonia and two per cent who developed neither disease. Moreover, methacholine inhalation (page 79) showed that 62 per cent of the children who suffered bronchiolitis and 45 per cent of the pneumonia group had hypersensitive airways.

RSV causes about three-quarters of bronchiolitis cases. Other viruses, including influenza, account for the rest. RSV is incredibly infectious – it infects half of all children by their first birthday, and by their third birthday every child has been infected. Fortunately, not every infection leads to bronchiolitis. In most cases the child recovers completely, and usually the wheeze is relatively short-lived.

Up to 75 per cent of infants with viral bronchiolitis develop wheezing. This falls to less than 50 per cent up to the age of five years, and to less than 25 per cent up to the age of ten years. Nevertheless, some children still show decreased lung function and increased reactivity 8–12 years later.

Some specialists suggest that bronchiolitis may predispose a child to asthma by establishing a long-standing inflammation in the lung. If this is the case, treating children suffering from bronchiolitis with steroids – drugs that reduce inflammation – should delay or prevent asthma. Preliminary studies suggest that nebulised steroids (page 130) can prevent wheezing. However, new studies currently underway must confirm these early findings before this treatment can be widely advocated.

Social deprivation

In parts of the country with good access to health care, few people die from asthma. Indeed, the risk of death among people with asthma may be no different to that among the general population. However, social deprivation increases the risk of developing asthma and makes a hospital admission more likely.

- Twice as many children in the deprived Bronx district of New York suffer from asthma than the average for the United States as a whole.
- In the UK, asthma is twice as common among the two lowest socioeconomic groups than in the highest two.
- A study in the West Midlands found that people over five years of age in the most deprived areas were nearly four times as likely to be admitted to hospital suffering from asthma than their more affluent neighbours.
- Moreover, poorer asthma sufferers were 2.5 times more likely to attend casualty rather than going to their GP. This may suggest that patients living in deprived areas feel that the primary health care system does not meet their needs and they will be treated more rapidly in hospital.

Certain asthma triggers are more common in socially deprived areas. We have already seen that the cockroach may be commoner in lower-income homes. Other factors may also contribute to an increased risk:

- housing is more likely to be damp and mouldy
- lower income groups are more likely to smoke
- lower income groups are less able to afford fresh fruits and vegetables
- pollution levels tend to be higher in deprived inner cities
- educational initiatives may not reach lower socioeconomic groups
- manual work may expose people to more occupational triggers than white-collar workers
- lower income groups may be unable to afford prescription charges – 48 per cent of asthma sufferers pay for their medicine, though prescriptions are free for children and for those on income support.

Why is asthma becoming more common?

Many asthma triggers have been around for centuries, so why is asthma becoming more common? It is unlikely that there is a single culprit. Several factors probably need to interact to account for the rise, including:

- increased levels of indoor allergens – especially the house dust mite and dander
- increased levels of outdoor air pollution, such as particulate pollution (page 41) and car exhaust fumes
- increased levels of indoor air pollution, such as gases released by gas cooker and heaters
- increased smoking during pregnancy
- more passive smoking
- changes in diet – especially a low intake of fresh fruit and vegetables containing the anti-oxidant vitamins and minerals (e.g. vitamins A, C and E, selenium and zinc) that mop up tissue-damaging free radicals, a product of the body's metabolism
- children are now less likely to contract childhood infections

than in the past. As a result, the immune system targets other organs – the so-called 'idling immune system' theory.

The asthma season

Asthma attacks tend to be more common at certain times of the year. Hospital admissions for asthma tend to peak in the autumn, and more than half of young adults with asthma report that their asthma follows a seasonal pattern.

- A study from Canada suggests that there is a fourfold increase in hospitalisations for asthma among pre-school children between July and October.
- Other studies report that asthma admissions peak between September and November.

The reason for this 'asthma season' is not fully understood. It probably arises from a number of causes, including climate, air pollution, the seasonal pattern in respiratory infections and variations in allergens borne by the wind (such as pollen and mould spores). Infections seem to be the main culprit, however. For example, the prevalence of acute bronchitis – which reliably indicates the rate of all respiratory infections – also rises during the autumn. The numbers of admissions for acute bronchitis and asthma tend to peak at the same time. These factors are exacerbated by the cold autumn air – cold air can be an asthma trigger. So the autumn asthma season reflects the allergen load (the number of allergens in the environment), individual sensitivity and climate.

Your own personal asthma season may be worse in the winter, spring or summer depending on your individual pattern of allergens. Therefore, people sensitive to tree pollen tend to develop symptoms in the spring, while those allergic to mould develop symptoms in the autumn. But some people are allergic to two or more allergens, so someone allergic to the house dust mite may suffer asthma throughout the year – but, as they are also sensitive to grass pollen, their asthma may worsen in the summer. Regularly checking lung function by monitoring your peak flow (page 73) allows you to identify your asthma season and take preventative steps. For example, increasing your dose of inhaled steroid for a couple of weeks before the season starts may prevent your condition worsening.

Asthma and family history

The link between genes and asthma first emerged following a shipwreck on the isolated Atlantic island of Tristan da Cunha. Three women among the original fifteen settlers suffered from asthma. Inbreeding was rife. Today, 30 per cent of the islanders have asthma.

We now know that many asthma sufferers report a family history of allergic disorders, including eczema and hay fever. There is a marked overlap between the three 'atopic' diseases: asthma, eczema and hay fever (allergic rhinitis), and indeed they share many trigger factors. For example, pollen, the house dust mite and animal fur can cause any, or all, of the conditions.

However, genes are just as important. For example:

- if neither parent suffers from an allergy, their child has a 15 per cent chance of developing an atopic condition
- if the mother is allergic, the risk is 40 per cent
- if both parents are allergic, the risk is 60 per cent
- if both parents have asthma rather than one of the other allergic diseases, the risk is over 80 per cent.

Moreover, atopy often emerges sooner among children with a family history of allergic disease. Forty-two per cent of children with two allergic parents develop an allergy within the first 18 months of life – twice the rate among children with only one allergic patient.

Studies of twins confirm the importance of genetic factors in asthma. If one twin suffers from asthma, the other is more likely to suffer from the disease than otherwise expected. Partly, of course, this could reflect their shared environment. Yet when identical twins are brought up in different homes, both twins are still at increased risk.

Why does allergic disease run in families?

Instead of inheriting a disease, the children of allergic parents inherit a tendency to produce high levels of the allergy antibody, immunoglobulin E (IgE). This leaves them vulnerable to developing an allergy. However, the way that this tendency expresses itself – as asthma, eczema or hay fever – depends on the allergens in the environment. Indeed, doctors believe that genes and environmental factors probably contribute equally to determining a child's IgE levels.

None of this means that you should blame yourself if your child develops asthma. Until we can choose our parents, we will not be able to choose our genes. It is worth bearing in mind that in other stages in our evolution, the genes responsible for asthma probably protected us from parasitic infections by ensuring high levels of IgE.

The three atopic diseases are becoming more common. A study carried out in Aberdeen measured the number of 8- to 13-year-olds suffering from hay fever, asthma and eczema in 1964 and then again in 1989. As the table shows, there has been a marked increase in the number of children suffering from these conditions. Part of the reason for the overlap lies the genetic basis of asthma and other atopic diseases.

Table 4: The rise in atopic disease 1964–1989

Illness or symptom	Percentage of children with the condition	
	1964	1989
Asthma	4.1	0.2
Wheeze	10.4	9.8
Shortness of breath	5.4	10.0
Hay fever	3.2	1.9
Eczema	5.3	12.0

The overlap with hay fever

Hay fever (allergic rhinitis) usually starts between the ages of eight and twenty, and tends to become less severe as people get older. Overall, maybe one in three children and adolescents suffer from the condition. There is a very marked overlap between asthma and hay fever: 20–25 per cent of patients with hay fever also suffer symptoms typical of asthma. A recent study suggested that three-quarters of people with asthma also suffer from the symptoms of hay fever.

The symptoms of hay fever include:

- nasal congestion – a blocked nose that is not relieved by blowing
- frequent sneezing

- a clear nasal discharge
- itching of the nose, mouth palate and throat
- conjunctival infection – itchy, sore and bloodshot eyes
- headache
- disturbed sleep and fatigue.

A wide variety of effective over-the-counter hay fever treatments are available from your pharmacist. If these fail, doctors can also prescribe a number of more potent hay fever treatments.

The overlap with eczema

Eczema is one of the most visible, unpleasant and disfiguring of diseases. People who have the condition endure dry, itchy, inflamed skin that can blister, weep, thicken and crack. Most children suffering from eczema first develop symptoms between the ages of six months and two years. They may be unable to sleep and make constant demands on their parents – which can leave the entire family tired and irritable. Like hay fever and asthma, atopic eczema is becoming more common.

The disease can be broadly divided into contact dermatitis and allergic eczema. Essentially, contact dermatitis is triggered by a chemical irritant; some children develop contact dermatitis which disappears after their parents change their brand of bubble bath or washing powder. Allergic eczema results from a hypersensitive immune system.

About 80 per cent of patients develop symptoms of eczema by their first birthday and 95 per cent within the first five years. Children with eczema are at least three times more likely to develop asthma than other children. Indeed, 40–80 per cent of children with eczema are treated for asthma at some time. Some specialists believe that given the appropriate conditions, almost all children with eczema may develop asthma. Unlike asthma, however, most children usually grow out of eczema. In some patients eczema has a tendency to recur, but about half of all children with eczema improve by school age and 90 per cent of cases resolve during adolescence.

A number of treatments are available for eczema. Adding emollients (oils) to the bath removes crusty skin scales and moisturises the skin. You can also apply emollients (creams) directly to the skin after a bath, or before swimming in a pool – chlorine tends to exacerbate eczema. If eczema does not respond to these simple measures in combination with allergen avoidance techniques (see **Chapter 8**), your GP can refer you to a dermatologist who can instigate more intensive treatment. Contact the National Eczema Society* for further information.

Asthma and anaphylactic shock

King Menes of Egypt died in 2641 BC after being stung by an insect. This was probably the first report of a death due to **anaphylaxis**, which is a severe reaction to allergens found in food or other agents. Since then numerous people have died after eating peanuts, taking certain medicines or being stung. One in every 3,000 people in hospital develops anaphylaxis, and it kills 3–9 per cent of all those affected. Anaphylaxis can kill remarkably rapidly. In 85 per cent of cases, the reaction occurs within 30 minutes of exposure to the allergen while in 96 per cent the reaction time is less than two hours.

A recent study suggests that one in seven deaths attributable to acute asthma may be caused by anaphylaxis – post-mortems carried out on people diagnosed as suffering from asthma revealed that the lungs of 15 per cent of the victims did not show the changes typical of asthma. The researchers believe that at least some of these deaths followed anaphylaxis. Ironically, some of these deaths may be entirely avoidable, since rapid diagnosis and prompt treatment with an injection of adrenaline (page 132) can save lives. Yet one test found that less than 40 per cent of doctors recognise the classic signs of anaphylaxis, some of which resemble asthma.

The signs of anaphylactic shock

Anaphylaxis occurs when allergens enter the bloodstream and cause a massive release of histamine. People who survive several anaphylactic attacks complain of an aura – a feeling of impeding doom or great peace – just before the onset of other signs. Symptoms caused by the rush of histamine in the body include bronchoconstriction, rashes and itching. The lips, tongue and larynx may swell, restricting breathing.

53

Besides increasing mucus production and triggering inflammation, the histamine explosion dilates blood vessels. If this happens throughout the body the blood pressure can fall to dangerously low levels – a condition known as hypotensive shock. Other problems may include the blood vessels becoming leaky, causing blood to seep into the vocal cords – this blocks the trachea and makes breathing difficult. In an emergency, a doctor may perform a tracheotomy (make a hole in the throat just below the Adam's apple) to release the blood and free the airway. Other signs of anaphylactic shock include:

- **cardiovascular system**: low blood pressure, shock, collapse, raised heart rate
- **eyes**: conjunctivitis, sneezing and tear production
- **gastrointestinal tract**: nausea and vomiting, diarrhoea, abdominal cramps or discomfort
- **mouth**: itching or a metallic taste in the mouth; swelling of the lips, face, tongue and throat.
- **nose**: congestion, swelling
- **respiratory tract**: wheeze, bronchoconstriction, asthma, choking, throat tightness
- **skin**: rash, hives, erythema (patchy inflammation of the skin), flushing, itching

Clearly, it is important to recognise the signs of anaphylaxis and seek medical treatment as quickly as possible. If you have had an anaphylactic attack in the past, consider carrying an adrenaline injection with you at all times. It could save your life. The Anaphylaxis Campaign★ offers further advice and support.

CHAPTER 3

THE PSYCHOLOGY OF ASTHMA

FOR many years, doctors regarded asthma as a psychosomatic illness. They believed that the characteristic breathlessness and wheezing were signs of emotional or mental distress, rather than the symptoms of a physical condition. Followers of the famous psychoanalyst, Sigmund Freud, argued that people with asthma were 'whining', 'obsessive', 'neurotic', 'complaining', 'lacking in self-confidence' and 'frequently depressed'. These elements were thought to make up the 'asthma personality'. Some doctors even suggested that people with asthma had a strong unexpressed dependency on their mothers. The wheezing was a suppressed cry.

Few theories have done so much harm. Asthma is not a disease of the mind; it is a disease of the lungs. Asthma is not caused by suppressed emotion; it is caused by inflammation. Asthma cannot be treated through psychotherapy; it can be treated with anti-inflammatories (**Chapter 5**). However, the idea that asthma has its roots in emotional disturbances meant that many people never brought their children forward for treatment, while some adults saw asthma as a sign of weakness. The misguided view that asthma's roots lay in the mind, rather than the lung, condemned patients to silent suffering and a mediocre quality of life – perhaps even death.

The psychological effects

Psychological and emotional factors do play an important role in asthma. That people with asthma may be obsessive, depressed and lacking in self-confidence is, perhaps, hardly surprising. Sufferers may become 'obsessive' about dusting or cleanliness if dust or dander triggers their asthma, for example. They may lack self-confidence because they worry that they will have an attack in public. They may become depressed if they suffer a serious attack and are unable to do things they used to. But psychological and emotional distress – although very real and common among people with asthma – tend to arise *because* of the asthma rather than being its cause.

Several studies suggest that certain personality traits increase the likelihood of developing symptoms. A study of 715 subjects, aged 22–44, found that anxious and depressed asthma sufferers were more likely to develop the following symptoms:

- wheeze
- waking breathless or with chest tightness
- attacks of breathlessness when resting
- attacks of breathlessness after activity.

Experiencing anxiety or depression does not influence lung function. So perhaps these patients' symptoms were due more to their state of mind than to their asthma.

The power of suggestion can, however, influence lung function, as shown by the results of an experiment using a placebo (a harmless salt solution that adult patients inhaled, believing it to contain an allergen):

- 19 out of 40 showed reduced lung function
- 12 patients developed symptoms.

According to some researchers, people who show marked bronchial hypersensitivity to methacholine challenge (page 79) tend to be more anxious than people who display a less dramatic response. This does not mean that anxiety causes asthma. Rather, it may reflect the emotional toll imposed by poorly controlled asthma.

In some ways, slight anxiety about asthma is a good thing. Mild anxiety acts as a mental spur, prodding us to change our lifestyle – the trick is to maintain a balance. Over-anxious people with asthma tend to have longer and more frequent episodes of hospitalisation, and use oral steroids more frequently, than less anxious people with the same severity of symptoms and lung function. On the other hand, too little anxiety can trigger a blatant disregard for symptoms that increases the risk of hospitalisation. But how can the mind affect asthma?

The mind–body link

Until relatively recently, most doctors treated diseases of the mind and body as separate. Even asylums for mental patients were built some distance away from general hospitals. However, over the last 20 years doctors have reconsidered the traditional split between mind and body. It is now clear that communication between the mind and the body runs both ways.

How the mind affects the immune system

We have already seen that the immune response underlying asthma (page 19) also protects us from invasion by foreign organisms – particularly parasites. Typically, when we encounter an allergen white blood cells are activated that release chemicals called inflammatory mediators. These can stimulate nerves in the lungs, causing asthmatic cough and other symptoms. The nerves also carry signals to the brain.

The brain feeds back to the immune system through nerves supplying the bone marrow, thymus gland, spleen, lymph nodes and other organs, increasing the production of white blood cells – the main line of defence against infection. This response is called 'nerve-mediated immunity' and is bolstered by the release of hormones from the pituitary and adrenal glands. The pituitary gland releases growth hormone and prolactin when the body is under stress. Both hormones profoundly influence the immune system's ability to fight infections: boosting it in the short-term; reducing its efficiency if exposure is prolonged. Short-term stress also increases the number and activity of natural killer cells – the white blood cells that destroy invading bacteria and viruses.

Scientists are now beginning to understand why excessive stress and some mental illnesses could directly worsen asthma. As described above, increased activity of natural killer cells and the hormonal surge protect us from infections after a possible injury. However, during chronic stress – stress that continues for long periods – levels of growth hormone, prolactin and natural killer cell activity decrease. This decline in the immune system's activity may have evolved to protect us from the risk of developing autoimmune disease (when the body produces antibodies that attack its own tissues). But the winding down of the body's defence system leaves us vulnerable to infection. Low levels of growth hormone, for example, seem to reduce white blood cell activity and inhibit antibody production: animals deprived of growth hormone are more likely to die after infection with salmonella and listeria.

In the same way, humans suffering severe stress or depression are more likely to be unable to fend off infections. Common diseases such as colds, influenza and respiratory infections, easily contracted when the immune system is at a low ebb, might also aggravate the condition of someone with asthma. (You could consider being vaccinated against influenza – see page 195.) It is therefore important to take steps to maintain good mental, as well as physical, health. For information about how to combat stress, see **Chapter 9**.

The brain's influence over the levels of hormones and blood cells in the body is involuntary. Yet the intimate relationship between the mind and the immune system provides startling proof of the way the former can influence the latter and *vice versa*.

Denial

In addition to feelings of anxiety and depression, denial is common among people with asthma. Denial is a mental self-defence technique – someone will employ it to avoid accepting the reality of their situation, even when faced with overwhelming evidence. Smokers may deny the damage that their addiction is doing, for example. Terminally ill patients may avoid facing facts until they can muster the emotional reserves to face the truth. And some people with asthma use denial to push the disease into their subconscious.

Denial is a powerful way to protect yourself from the ravages of depression and anxiety. Indeed, patients not obviously suffering from psychiatric disease who suffer near-fatal asthma attacks are more likely to enter denial than those who suffer from depression and anxiety. Denial may form part of the legacy of a severe asthma attack that lingers long after the patient returns home. One survey suggests that almost 60 per cent of people who experience near-fatal asthma attacks show high levels of denial – despite the severity of their condition. Often, these patients play down their condition before the attack. But a brush with death sends them even further into denial. This undermines their chances of controlling their asthma in the future. There are also social reasons why patients enter denial. Culturally, we value health and fitness. Denial helps patients to feel they are able to 'fit in' with our social norms.

Why not everyone follows the rules

Though asthma can be life-threatening and ruin patients' quality of life, 30–50 per cent of people with asthma do not take their medication as instructed by their doctor. This refusal – or inability – to follow medical advice is called **poor compliance**. As we will see in **Chapter 5**, asthma drugs that control the underlying inflammation must be taken regularly to prevent acute attacks. Not taking your anti-inflammatories leaves you vulnerable to an attack. Yet at one medical practice in Liverpool, almost half the patients did not collect enough inhalers to take even 50 per cent of their recommended doses of anti-inflammatories. Whatever the reason, these people showed poor compliance. Indeed, no one should think themself exempt – everyone is vulnerable to the hazards of disregarding treatment, irrespective of age, sex, education, economic status, or the frequency and severity of symptoms.

Your mental state may undermine compliance. One study measured anxiety, depression and interpersonal problems among 102 adults with asthma, for example.

Doctors interviewed patients about their attitudes towards self-care, social support, treatment and acceptance of medical authority. A computerised system assessed the patients' compliance as they used asthma medication over 12 weeks.

- 37 people took less than 70 per cent of the prescribed dose, or omitted doses for one week. These patients were more likely to suffer from depression and anxiety.

- The patients' reports of themselves – and even the clinicians' impressions – did not accurately predict who would follow treatment and who would not.

Similarly, in another study only 10 out of 39 subjects used inhaled drugs correctly. Patients who used their inhalers arbitrarily tended to have higher levels of general anxiety and were less able to recognise the first symptoms of an imminent asthma attack.

As many as 60 per cent of people with asthma cannot tell when their lung function takes a turn for the worse. Indeed, patients with the most severe asthma, the most extensive airway obstruction and the greatest bronchial hypersensitivity most frequently underestimate the severity of their airway obstruction. Their lungs – or perhaps the part of the brain that senses changes in lung function – seem to adapt to a level of obstruction that would provoke symptoms in someone with milder asthma. In addition, many people adapt their lifestyle to fit their symptoms: if you feel a bit breathless you might walk more slowly so as not to feel uncomfortable, for instance. It is clear that understanding and compliance can improve only if treatment is based on objective measurements of airway obstruction – such as peak flow (page 72) – rather than subjective experience of symptoms. In other words, you should rely on your peak flow chart rather than how you think you feel.

Other reasons for non-compliance

There are several other reasons why people with asthma may not follow their doctors' instructions.

Age and ability

Asthma in the elderly (see pages 175–9) often has to be managed against a background of other conditions, such as arthritis and poor vision. An elderly person's ability to cope with inhaler treatment is determined by his or her mental state and the severity of other diseases, rather than age. Between 15 and 20 per cent of the over-80s show signs of mental impairment, but an elderly person who has retained normal mental abilities and does not have joint disease can manage just as well as a younger patient.

In the same way, young people with learning disabilities may be unable to use an inhaler. Sometimes, parents may not understand how to treat their child or know how the inhaler works.

Poor inhaler technique

Pressured metered dose inhalers are the commonest way of delivering drugs for asthma. However, only about half of patients use these correctly – a problem that often goes unrecognised. Another option is to switch to another easier-to-use device, such as a dry powder inhaler. **Chapter 5** describes inhaler devices and correct technique.

A dislike of medication

About 28 per cent of people dislike taking inhaled steroids and up to 50 per cent worry about side-effects – see **Chapter 5** – even though inhaled steroids are relatively safe (the risks of uncontrolled asthma are far more serious). So these people may, albeit unconsciously, become lax about taking their drugs. Some other anti-inflammatories have to be taken four times a day, which may be inconvenient and make life difficult for parents who cannot supervise their child's medication while he or she is at school.

Poor understanding

Asthma treatment works on two levels. Bronchodilators alleviate acute asthma by opening the airways, but allow the underlying inflammation to continue – just papering over the cracks, in effect. This is why doctors also prescribe an anti-inflammatory to control the underlying inflammation.

A European survey suggests that 23 per cent of people with moderate asthma and 19 per cent with severe asthma do not understand that anti-inflammatory medication prevents asthma symptoms. In some ways, this could be the fault of the doctors who do not clearly explain the reason for prescribing both drugs. Yet understanding the difference between bronchodilators and anti-inflammatories is essential if patients are to derive the most benefit from their treatment. **Chapter 5** discusses in more detail the drugs used to treat asthma.

The stress of adolescent asthma

The stress of asthma and pressures to fit in are especially marked among adolescents. Adolescence is stressful enough without the added burden of asthma. Perhaps as a result, adolescents with asthma are more likely to abuse alcohol and smoke than those without asthma:

- 46 per cent of asthmatic Australian 15-year-olds drink at least once weekly, compared to 34 per cent of their peers who don't have asthma
- 25 per cent smoke, compared to 11 per cent of those without asthma.

Teenagers with asthma are also roughly twice as likely to develop psychosomatic symptoms – such as feeling dizzy and experiencing headaches and backache – than their peers without asthma. These conditions are probably at least partly rooted in the mind. Adolescents who have asthma are also more likely to feel lonely, low and depressed, generally unhappy, irritable, worried about below-average school performance and unable to sleep.

Young people with asthma are particularly vulnerable, so it is important that they are able to express their feelings and vent their anger and frustrations. For more information see 'The three ages of asthma', page 162.

Stress in the family

Though asthma can bring people together in concern over a loved one, it can be emotionally draining for a sufferer's family. If the person affected is a child, the parents will have to learn how to cope with his or her medication and be prepared to deal with an acute asthma attack (see page 157 for what to do). A diagnosis of asthma can seem a daunting sentence for both the sufferer and their relatives. However, other factors can exacerbate the stress.

For example, people with asthma may become over-dependent on relatives and medical staff – if they have endured a near-fatal asthma attack they might try to minimise the effect of the disease, perhaps through denial (see above). Family members, meanwhile, may try to over-protect the sufferer – especially if they have witnessed him or her having a severe attack. The patient, perhaps fortunately, usually forgets. On the patient's return from hospital, relatives may repress their anger and continue to over-involve themselves in his or her welfare, inevitably causing stress and tension. So it is important to bolster the family's, as well as the patient's, stress defences. **Chapter 9** describes various therapies that relieve stress, as well as helping asthma.

Doctors acknowledge the importance of psychological and social factors in asthma, though few tackle them. Prompt diagnosis and effective treatment, allied with greater understanding, could work wonders in averting misapprehension, fear and unecessary suffering. The next chapter deals with the diagnosis of asthma.

CHAPTER 4

IS IT ASTHMA OR NOT?

You might expect that doctors would find a condition as common as asthma easy to diagnose. In fact, diagnosis often proves difficult. Is your cough caused by asthma or a cold? Are you breathless because you are unfit or because you have asthma? Is your child wheezing because he or she has picked up a virus or because it is the first sign of asthma? Certain diseases produce symptoms very similar to asthma – bronchiolitis, for example, causes coughing, wheezing and swelling of the airways – and not all wheezes, coughs and complaints of breathlessness are signs of asthma.

To make matters worse, asthma is an emotive word. Most children recover completely from mild respiratory infections. This clearly is not the case with asthma. Sufferers and their parents fear they will no longer be able to live a normal life. They worry that they may even die.

Diagnosing asthma is also a loaded issue for doctors. Asthma is often a long-term condition and a child with asthma needs regular supervision. Parents understandably worry, and may call out the doctor in the middle of the night. As a result, many doctors are reluctant to diagnose asthma in children. They may label persistent childhood wheeze as 'wheezy bronchitis'.

Asthma is difficult to diagnose accurately. If you or your child shows mild signs of asthma, your GP may make a best guess based on the history and symptoms and prescribe a course of anti-inflammatories and bronchodilators (see **Chapter 5**). This 'suck-it-and-see' approach – properly called a therapeutic trial – works on the principle that if the drugs are effective, you have the disease. If not, the doctor reconsiders the diagnosis.

To make things more difficult for physicians, there is no definitive diagnostic test for asthma. If a doctor thinks you are suffering from an infection, he or she can send a sample to a microbiology lab to determine the bacteria responsible and the most appropriate antibiotic to prescribe. But used alone, none of the tests described in this chapter can prove without doubt that you have asthma. As a result, you may undergo a round of examinations.

In many cases, doctors will make a diagnosis based on your symptoms, history and peak flow measurements (page 72). However, if you are not responding as well as expected, you may be referred to a specialist who will perform some more advanced tests. Some tests can determine the allergen or trigger that provokes your asthma – though as will be shown later, testing positive to a particular allergen does not necessarily mean that it is responsible for your asthma. Indeed, as many as 40 per cent of the general population test positive to common allergens, yet not all these people develop atopic (allergic) disease – asthma, hay fever or eczema (see **Chapter 2**).

This chapter looks at some of the tests that you might undergo to confirm your doctor's suspicions; to monitor your response to treatment; and to uncover the triggers that might be responsible.

The asthma mimics

A number of lung diseases cause symptoms similar to the hallmarks of asthma – twitchy airways, excessive mucus production and inflamed bronchi.

Chronic obstructive pulmonary disease (COPD)

Chronic obstructive pulmonary disease (COPD) covers a multitude of respiratory diseases and describes any long-standing obstructive disease affecting the lung, although most doctors associate it with chronic bronchitis or emphysema. The description 'obstructive pulmonary' refers to the blocked airways characteristic of the illness. COPD is common: some 10–15 per cent of male smokers aged 55–64 develop the condition.

Chronic bronchitis
Chronic bronchitis is a long-lasting inflammatory disease, usually

caused by smoking. The inflammation in chronic bronchitis damages the airways, producing persistent cough and phlegm. The mucus tends to trap bacteria or viruses, leading to periodic infections – a condition called acute bronchitis. Lung damage tends to be more extensive in chronic bronchitis than in asthma, as the inflammation is combined with the effects of smoking. As a result, the airway obstruction is generally less reversible than the brochoconstriction characteristic of asthma.

Consequently, if asthma medication nearly completely reverses the airway obstruction, the doctor is likely to assume that the patient has asthma. If there is little change, he or she may presume that the patient has COPD. COPD and asthma can overlap, however. Most COPD patients show improved lung function after using bronchodilators. They become less breathless and are better able to exercise. As a result, doctors sometimes confuse asthma and COPD, especially among middle-aged and elderly smokers.

Croup

Croup is a common childhood disease that may seem similar to asthma. Caused by a virus, it tends to affect the under-fives – usually during the autumn and winter.

Children develop:

- cold-like symptoms
- hoarse voice
- barking cough
- wheeziness on inhalation (called 'stridor')
- mild breathing problems
- mild fever (usually not above 38°C).

Croup usually improves within a week, although it may recur.

Cystic fibrosis

Cystic fibrosis is a serious disease caused by an abnormal gene – although sufferers need to inherit two copies (one from the mother and one from the father) before they develop symptoms. As a result of this genetic defect, the lung produces copious amounts of thick, sticky mucus. This provides the ideal breeding ground for bacteria, and the person with the condition is vulnerable to repeated lung infections.

However, the disease also affects the pancreas and other glands, including those in the skin. As a result, people with cystic fibrosis excrete excessive amounts of sodium in their sweat, so a sweat test can detect most cases. Treatment is improving – the average life expectancy is now 29 years, compared to two years 30 years ago. Most specialists agree that life expectancy will continue to improve.

Gastro-oesophageal reflux

People with asthma are some three times more likely to suffer from gastro-oesophageal reflux than those without the condition. The link with gastro-oesophageal reflux is not clear, although it may be particularly pronounced among people with nocturnal asthma. Asthma sufferers with gastro-oesophageal reflux may regurgitate small amounts of stomach acid into their mouth and into their trachea (windpipe). Others may regurgitate just into the oesophagus (food pipe), where the acid burns the delicate lining, stimulating the nerves. Both of these can exacerbate asthma. Factors that may be responsible for someone developing the condition include:

- stress – tension increases the risk of developing gastro-oesophageal reflux
- treatment – e.g. theophylline (page 116) relaxes the muscles that prevent the acid from regurgitating. Steroid tablets can cause indigestion and ulcers.

If you develop gastro-oesophageal reflux, try taking an antacid, H2 antagonist or other indigestion remedy available from your chemist, or consult your GP. You should also cut down on fatty food and alcohol and eat smaller, more frequent meals. Smoking also causes gastro-oesophageal reflux – another good reason to quit.

If you think your steroid tablets are giving you indigestion, consult your GP.

Heart disease

Some types of heart disease mimic asthma, making diagnosis especially difficult among elderly people. Congestive heart failure, which can develop after a heart attack, can cause similar symptoms to asthma.

During a heart attack, parts of the heart muscle are starved of oxygen and die. The heart muscles weaken as a result, and the heart pumps blood less efficiently. Subsequently, fluid pools in the lung (pulmonary oedema) inhibiting the transfer of oxygen. Patients with pulmonary oedema often develop symptoms similar to those of nocturnal asthma (page 25), including wheezing and breathlessness. Indeed, pulmonary oedema was once known as 'cardiac asthma'. In cases of doubt a chest X-ray usually resolves the diagnosis.

Asthma and heart disease are common conditions, and some people develop both. The prospects for patients with both diseases are far worse than for someone with just one complaint.

Obliterative bronchiolitis

Obliterative bronchiolitis arises when the small bronchi are destroyed. Some people with rheumatoid arthritis develop it when inflammation spills over from the joints and begins attacking the lungs: the symptoms closely mimic asthma. Fortunately, obliterative bronchiolitis is rare (do not confuse this with the childhood infection).

Psychological conditions

Asthma is not caused by nerves, although stress can exacerbate asthma (see **Chapter 3**). Certain psychological conditions can mimic the symptoms of asthma, however.

Psychogenic vocal cord dysfunction
Sufferers of this rare condition, also called psychogenic stridor, develop asthma-like symptoms. The steroids that doctors may prescribe are, not surprisingly, ineffective – patients are therefore assumed to be resistant to steroids, and may be given more powerful drugs.

Psychogenic vocal cord dysfunction is an expression of stress, rather than a sign of asthma. By displaying symptoms, the patient is able to avoid confronting tense situations in the family or elsewhere. Sufferers are usually women and the condition is found most often in societies with rigidly defined roles: the Arabic community, for example.

The condition may accompany genuine asthma: people with asthma who get anxious may subconsciously exaggerate their asthma by 'glottic wheezing'.

Hyperventilation (over-breathing) can also make you seem breathless. Hyperventilation is a common reaction to stress and may also be a sign of an asthma attack, so separating the two can prove difficult.

Affective hypersensitivity

In some patients, 'affective hypersensitivity' can confuse diagnosis. These people have *bona fide* asthma. Their condition is originally triggered by a specific allergen – flower pollen, say. But later, non-specific smells, such as a perfume with the scent of roses, begin to trigger symptoms. Eventually, merely thinking about the trigger is enough – even a fleeting glimpse of a bouquet of plastic flowers can trigger an asthma attack.

Some researchers believe that some asthma attacks among patients who develop affective hypersensitivity are a form of non-verbal communication. But this does not mean the asthma has its roots in the mind. Instead, the genuine allergic symptoms come first and the mind uses the disease as a way to express its distress.

Psychogenic cough

Psychogenic cough is usually dry or throaty and ranges from a simple clearing of the throat to a coughing fit lasting several minutes. Often, teenagers develop the condition following an infection or a mild asthma attack. The cough is likely to disappear during sleep or when the child is distracted. Sufferers frequently have a history of stomach pains, headaches, nightmares and other psychosomatic diseases as a child – although teenagers with the condition usually appear intelligent, compulsive and eager to please.

The cough can become the focus of the family's life. Not surprisingly, parents may become tired and irritable, whereas the teenager will seem worn out but otherwise well. In these cases, the family may benefit from relaxation techniques (**Chapter 9**). Counselling may also help uncover the cause of the conflict – your GP may be able to suggest a good local counsellor. Alternatively, contact the British Association for Counselling.★ In many cases, the teenager also suffers from true asthma and disentangling the physical and psychological causes can prove difficult.

Difficulties in diagnosing children

Some specific problems are associated with the diagnosis of asthma in children.

Younger children, especially those under five years of age, may find some of the tests used for asthma – such as spirometry or using a peak flow meter (described later in this chapter) – difficult to perform. As we will see in **Chapter 6**, asthma treatment should be tailored to the seriousness of the patient's symptoms. Since testing many children is fruitless, doctors have to rely on their clinical acumen to decide whether they have asthma. Severe asthma is somewhat easier to recognise: a history of frequent trips to the local casualty unit is usually sufficient for the GP to diagnose severe asthma.

The problem with this approach is that the severity of the underlying inflammation may not translate into symptoms. Moreover, in many children coughing may be the main – or only – symptom of asthma. In addition, some children cough and wheeze in the night without waking their parents, who may not identify the warning signs.

You can take steps to help your doctor assess the severity of your child's asthma:

- Keep a diary recording the number of times that your child wakes during the night. (Note that a 'baby monitor' may not be much help, however. By amplifying every stirring, it may cause you to come rushing into the room only to find your child sleeping soundly.)
- It is important to note any possible triggers – e.g. exercise or stroking the cat.
- School absences may be a poor indicator of the severity of asthma. Rather, the number of days that a child skips school could be a better marker of his or her parents' anxiety. For example, the parents of a child who goes to a school where the teachers insist on locking the inhalers away may be more likely to allow him or her to skip school than the parents of a child

attending a school with a sensible asthma policy. And, of course, it is harder to stay at home if both parents go out to work.

- Parents may have very different perceptions of a child's symptoms – e.g. one may be generally unconcerned, the other distressed by every cough. This difference is even more marked when the parents are separated or divorced.

- You could keep a diary of your child's symptoms, so that you will be less reliant on fallible memory. This will also provide evidence with which to approach your GP if he or she is reluctant to diagnose asthma.

Lung function tests

Lung function or 'pulmonary' tests are widely used: to diagnose asthma; to assess the severity of symptoms; and to monitor response to treatment. They give doctors a clearer picture of your condition. Each test provides different information about lung function and, therefore, the severity of your asthma. Doctors focus on three measurements: peak expiratory flow rate, measured by a **peak flow meter**, and forced expiratory volume (FEV1) and forced vital capacity (FVC), which are measured by a **spirograph** (see below).

Lung function measurements vary according to your sex, fitness, age and build, as well as the severity of your asthma and the effectiveness of your treatment. Environmental factors, such as whether you are exposed to smoking on a day-to-day basis, can also be significant. So peak expiratory flow rate will be higher in a 20-year-old male jogger than in his 60-year-old arthritic grandmother, irrespective of any lung disease. As a result, lung function tests are often expressed as a percentage of the predicted average value for your sex and age group and can also be measured against your personal best. If you are within 80 per cent of your predicted average value, doctors regard your lung function as 'normal'. A value of 20 or even 60 per cent of your predicted value would suggest you are suffering from a lung disease.

The values of people who do not have asthma show considerable variation, however. A vital capacity of one litre below the average value could be due to either lung disease or natural variation.

As a result, doctors also take account of other factors – such as symptoms – when evaluating the results of lung function tests.

Peak flow

Peak flow monitoring is the most widely used lung function test. Peak expiratory flow meters, more commonly called peak flow meters, measure **peak expiratory flow rate**. This is the maximum flow rate of expired air during expiration, i.e. how fast you exhale. Peak flow meters are small enough to keep at home and are easy to use. Measuring peak flow allows doctors to assess the severity of your asthma – most accurately by comparing readings against your personal best, though it can also be calculated according to the following criteria:

- healthy people show a peak flow of 400–600 litres per minute
- people with asthma show a peak flow of 200–400 litres per minute
- in severe asthma attacks, peak flow can fall to 100 litres per minute.

Moreover, the morning and evening peak flow readings of people with asthma tend to show a greater variation than the readings of those without asthma:

- in people without asthma, the difference between morning and evening peak flow is less than 15 per cent
- in people with asthma, peak flow varies by over 20 per cent during the day
- symptoms do not usually emerge until peak flow falls by 25 per cent.

The diagram opposite plots peak flow readings. The 'saw tooth' pattern strongly indicates that you are suffering from asthma.

An early warning system for people with asthma

You cannot rely on symptoms alone to predict when you are likely to have an asthma attack. By the time you begin to wheeze, the inflammation is probably quite intense. As many as 60 per cent of people with asthma fail to recognise worsening symptoms, and ironically patients with severe asthma often have the worst perception of the

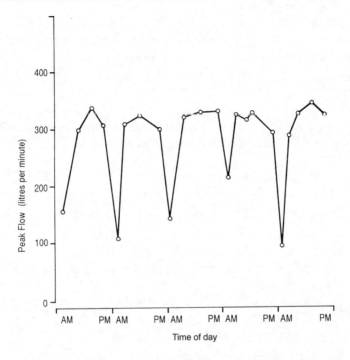

Figure 4   The 'saw tooth' peak flow pattern typical of asthma

severity of their airway obstruction. They seem to adapt to levels of obstruction that would provoke symptoms in someone with milder asthma, and alter their lifestyle to suit their symptoms (e.g. walking more slowly if breathless). In other words, you need an objective measure of lung function in order to take steps to prevent an attack.

Regularly monitoring your peak flow provides an early warning system that can detect deteriorating asthma, especially in adults. Peak flow increases when your condition is well controlled and declines when your airways narrow in response to a flare-up of the underlying inflammation. Doctors aim to maintain asthma patients' peak flow to within 20 per cent of that of people without asthma of the same age, height and sex, or within the same percentage of the patient's personal best. They also try to ensure that your values are stable from day to day and show little difference between morning and evening peak flow – the less variation between the two, the better the control. As a result, regular self-monitoring is vital to ensure that your asthma is optimally controlled (see 'How to use a peak flow meter', below).

Peak flow may decline by at least 25 per cent before you begin to show symptoms. If your peak flow falls by 20 per cent, your doctor may suggest increasing your dose of anti-inflammatory. As you are controlling your asthma at an early stage – even before symptoms emerge – you are more likely to be able to control the inflammation with low-dose inhaled steroids, rather than high-dose or oral steroids, which carry an increased risk of side-effects (see page 96). **Chapter 6** discusses self-management plans in more detail.

How to use a peak flow meter

Most people over the age of 5–7 can learn to use a peak flow meter. The technique is simple:

- check that the pointer is at zero
- sit upright or stand and lift your head
- hold the meter horizontally, keeping your fingers away from the pointer
- put the mouthpiece between your lips
- blow out as hard and quickly as you can
- note the reading, rest the pointer and begin again
- after three readings, note the highest reading on the chart.

Some doctors believe that you should regularly change your peak flow meter – research suggests that about a third of peak flow meters over a year old are inaccurate. You should wash your peak flow meter according to the manufacturer's instructions. Following these instructions and keeping your meter in a safe place where it cannot be damaged should extend its active life.

Other uses of peak flow

Peak flow meters can also help diagnose the cause of your asthma. For example, taking peak flow rate measurements every two hours while recording your activities for two weeks at work, and during a week off, may help diagnose occupational asthma (page 43). Analysing the readings may make it possible to pinpoint certain situations or agents that are making your condition worse. Peak flow meters can also help diagnose exercise-induced asthma (page 31).

In the same way, if you react to an asthma trigger a peak flow meter could highlight your susceptiblity. Peak flow declines over one hour after exposure to an allergen, e.g. cat dander, though the decline in peak flow tends to be slower if you have contracted a virus.

The problems with peak flow

Regularly measuring peak flow is undoubtedly important. However, peak flow has four main limitations.

- There is a danger that you could become over-reliant on your peak flow measurement. Some studies suggest that peak flow monitoring may not detect some asthma attacks, even if the patients' symptoms are severe enough to warrant oral steroids. The problem is that peak flow is not the only factor to influence symptom severity. Some patients do not develop symptoms at low peak flow levels, while others report symptoms at levels close to those predicted. Moreover, the level of breathlessness that patients show at any particular peak flow value varies widely. So you need to keep a note of night-time waking and how often you use your bronchodilator as well as peak flow.

- As you recover from a severe asthma attack, symptoms tend to disappear when peak flow reaches two-thirds of predicted values. However, the bronchi may still be hyper-responsive (twitchy) and it is important to continue your high dose of inhaled or oral steroids for the recommended time (just as it is imperative to complete a course of antibiotics). Reduce the dose of your steroids too quickly and the inflammation can flare up.

- Using a peak flow meter can be embarrassing for some older people. The effort to exhale as fast as possible can, if you have a weak bladder, lead to a small amount of urine leaking. If you find that this is a problem, and you are too embarrassed to use the meter in front of the nurse or doctor, you could go to the toilet before using the peak flow meter, or ask to measure your peak flow in another room.

- Just as patients do not always comply with treatment (see 'Why not everyone follows the rules', **Chapter 3**), they may not always follow the recommended guidelines for peak flow measurements. Not surprisingly, patients are most motivated when they feel ill and when they are recovering from an attack, provided denial is not a problem. Studies suggest that only 35 per cent of people monitor peak flow more than once a week when their asthma is well controlled, compared to the 81 per cent who do so during a period of deterioration.

In other words, you should not rely on peak flow alone. Provided you remember these limitations, there is no better alternative to provide you with an insight into the state of your asthma. Regular measurements can help you control your asthma – especially as part of a self-management plan (**Chapter 6**).

Spirometry

A spirograph offers another measurement of airway obstruction and helps confirm a diagnosis of asthma. Rather than measuring the patient's peak flow, the spirograph records airflow against time. As the subject breathes out, the volume of air exhaled is initially rapid but then slows down, before reaching a plateau. Doctors derive two measures from this:

- **forced expiratory volume in one second (FEV1)** – the volume of air expelled in one second
- **forced vital capacity (FVC)** – the volume attained when the patient breathes out until no further air can be expelled.

The diagram opposite shows tracings from a spirometer comparing values of an asthma patient and someone without asthma.

Healthy people take about four seconds to expel a full breath, discharging about three-quarters of their breath during the first second – an FEV1 of 70 per cent. Any condition that reduces vital capacity lowers FEV1, and the reduction is most marked when the airways are obstructed. The FEV1 of someone with asthma or a similar condition therefore falls to 50, or even 20 per cent. People with asthma can also take longer to expel all the air. The diagram shows tracings from a spirometer, comparing the values of an asthma patient and someone without asthma.

A large number of diseases can reduce vital capacity. They include fibrosis, muscle weakness and chest deformity. Since asthma and other conditions that cause airway obstruction tend to limit the rate of airflow, a fall in vital capacity is almost inevitable.

Bronchial reversibility

You may sometimes be asked to perform a bronchial reversibility test. As you will remember from **Chapter 1**, bronchoconstriction is reversible. Some doctors therefore measure your peak flow

Figure 5   FEV1 and FVC in people with and without asthma

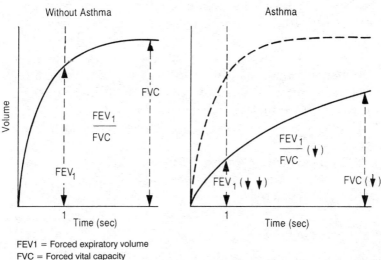

FEV1 = Forced expiratory volume
FVC = Forced vital capacity

before, and several minutes after, a puff of inhaled bronchodilator. If your peak flow improves by 15 per cent or more, you may have asthma. Most people with asthma show at least a 15 per cent increase in airflow during a bronchial reversibility test.

However, this method is not infallible. About a quarter of people with respiratory tract infections show a large, reversible increase in lung function when tested in this way. This reflects the inflammation triggered by the infection, not the presence of asthma. In addition, not all adults respond immediately to a reversibility test, particularly those with late-onset asthma. A negative bronchodilator response does not exclude asthma, but might indicate the need for a steroid trial – more proof of the importance of not relying on a single test for asthma.

Allergen tests

Often, finding the trigger of the asthma is a higher priority for patients than doctors. However, in many cases identifying the allergen does not change the treatment prescribed. There are exceptions – most notably in occupational asthma and aspirin-induced asthma – yet doctors often argue that even if the allergen is identified, relatively little can be done. It is one thing to know that you are allergic to grass pollen, but it is quite another to avoid it.

However, if you know you are allergic to pollen or the house dust mite there are a number of self-help steps that you can take (many of which are described in **Chapter 8**). A large number of people, often misguidedly, believe that their asthma is caused by food allergies – in this case dietary challenge tests may help (see page 81).

Don't underestimate the psychological benefits of putting your mind at rest. The following tests may indicate that a specific trigger could be responsible.

Skin prick testing

Although it is over 100 years old and despite of the arrival of newer, high-tech tests (described below), the skin prick test remains the most widely used method to determine possible allergens among people with asthma. Doctors have refined the technique over the last century. However, the basic principle remains the same: to get some of the suspected allergen under the skin and record what happens.

- The doctor or, more usually, nurse applies a drop of the test allergen to the surface of the skin – usually on the inside of the forearm. This allows a number of possible allergens to be tested.
- A lancet is then placed into the drop and pressed into the skin. The skin is then pressed with a soft tissue to help absorption.
- If you are 'sensitive' to the test allergen, the skin develops a smooth, raised lump known as a weal. This will usually be surrounded by a reddish flush, and may itch. After about 15 minutes, the intensity of the response is assessed by measuring the size of the weal.
- Taking antihistamines may affect the results of the test.

A skin reaction does not guarantee that the allergen is responsible for your asthma. Indeed, about 40 per cent of people without asthma react to one or more common allergens on skin testing. As a result, skin prick tests can only implicate possible suspects – they cannot prove that the allergen actually causes the symptoms. However, inhaling the allergen may offer further evidence (see below).

Inhalation challenge tests

As noted earlier, a number of factors – from cold air to chemicals and cat fur – can trigger an asthma attack in sensitive people. Skin prick tests may suggest a culprit, but the best way to assess whether a trigger is responsible is to expose the lungs to the suspected allergen and see whether lung function falls – a technique known as broncho-provocation, or inhalation challenge. This sounds dangerous, but accidents rarely occur in a carefully controlled hospital setting. During the test, the patient sits in a sealed chamber into which a quantity of the allergen is introduced. He or she then breathes in the agent. Should the patient suffer anaphylactic shock, the physician can step in with an injection of adrenaline to relieve the symptoms.

Doctors using inhalation challenge techniques employ three main methods of assessing airway responsiveness: histamine or methacholine challenge, non-allergic triggers and specific triggers (including allergens and occupational chemicals).

Histamine or methacholine challenge

Almost all asthma sufferers are hypersensitive to histamine and methacholine, which are non-allergenic chemicals – healthy people either do not react to these stimuli, or show only a mild response. In asthma sufferers, the drugs act directly on the muscles surrounding the bronchi, causing the airways to contract. After exposing the patient to histamine or methacholine in inhalation challenge, doctors assess the extent of bronchoconstriction using the lung function tests (see pages 71–77). Usually, doctors note what dose of histamine or methacholine will cause a 20 per cent reduction in the patient's FEV1 or peak flow.

People with severe asthma are adversely affected by weaker doses than people with moderate asthma, while the latter react at lower doses than people with mild asthma and those without asthma. People without asthma may not show even a 20 per cent reduction in FEV1 following exposure to the drugs.

There are a number of problems associated with histamine or methacholine challenge.

- Resting lung function, bronchodilator use, respiratory infections, recent acute asthma attacks and the time of day can all influence bronchoconstriction.
- Some people – e.g. those with an FEV1 less than 60 per cent of the predicted value – cannot perform histamine or methacholine challenge.
- A few people with asthma show normal responses to histamine or methacholine challenge; conversely in rare cases people without asthma may respond to the drugs.
- Histamine and methacholine challenge cannot necessarily predict symptom severity, diurnal variation or peak flow.

Non-allergic triggers

Other provocation tests use non-allergic triggers, such as exercise, hyperventilation and a fine spray of saline (salt solution) to assess bronchial hypersensitivity. People without asthma show a reduction of less than 10 per cent in FEV1 following exposure to these non-allergic triggers. The effect on lung function among people with asthma is more marked.

The drawbacks of this approach are that some patients are unable to exercise, and asthma sufferers often fail to respond predictably to exercise testing. Hyperventilation (rapid breathing) and inhaling a fine saline spray offer more consistent alternatives. However, it is not entirely certain how accurately results from any of these provocation tests reflect the underlying inflammation or severity of symptoms in someone with asthma.

Specific trigger tests

Doctors may also use inhalation tests to assess a patient's response to specific triggers or allergens. These tests are performed in hospital and provide important insights to the nature of asthma. Challenge tests are useful in diagnosing certain cases of occupational asthma (page 43) and aspirin-sensitive asthma (page 37).

- Patients suspected of suffering from aspirin-sensitive asthma might inhale a mist of soluble aspirin. Sensitive patients tend to react within 30–60 minutes.
- In other tests, some patients actually take aspirin tablets,

though the effects are more difficult to control. It is easy to stop someone breathing in a chemical; rather harder to remove a tablet from the body.

- Another method involves applying aspirin to the inside of the nose; symptoms usually occur after 15–30 minutes.

Inhalation tests for specific triggers have their limitations, however. Unlike skin prick testing, assessing a wide range of possible allergens is impracticable. Moreover, the test environment is somewhat artificial – contact with the allergen is brief rather than prolonged. In a provocation test, the patient may be exposed to an intense burst of pollen, rather than encountering it throughout the season. If skin prick tests have already shown that you test positive to, say, the house dust mite, it is doubtful whether further confirmation of this would alter the way you deal with the problem.

A fundamental problem with provocation tests is that almost everyone with twitchy airways responds to provocation. This does not necessarily mean that the patient has asthma. For example, smokers have hyper-reactive bronchi, as do people suffering from acute bronchitis. So while provocation tests can provide some insights, additional tests are also needed.

Dietary challenge tests

Dietary challenge tests were devised to help assess suspected food allergies. The following method is one of many programmes that can be adopted:

- you exclude suspect foods from your diet for 5–8 weeks
- one of the suspect foods is reintroduced, mixed with herbs and oils to disguise the flavour. You note the severity and frequency of the symptoms
- at some point, the doctor may also introduce a placebo – the herbs and oils without the specific allergen
- you – and ideally your doctor – do not know whether you have received the placebo or the allergen. If you react to the placebo, food is unlikely to be the cause of the symptoms
- dietary measures are combined with peak flow and spirometry tests.

More commonly, patients will follow an exclusion diet. As the name suggests, you ban the suspect food from your diet – this is easy if the trigger is shellfish, rather harder if it is dairy products. During the exclusion period you measure your peak flow before and during the diet. About ten days' exclusion should usually be enough to pinpoint the culprit. However, if suspicions prove wrong, finding the suspect food can take months.

Alternatively, some asthma sufferers exclude everything from their diet apart from a few bland foods. They then gradually reintroduce a normal diet, noting the response as they become reacquainted with various foods. This type of exclusion diet should be performed only under the supervision of a qualified dietician. See **Chapter 7** for more information about diet in pregnancy, food allergies and supervising your child's diet.

Other tests

Doctors may use a number of other tests to clarify a diagnosis of asthma.

- Coughing is a symptom of a number of respiratory diseases, including lung cancer. If you have problems with coughing, you may undergo a chest X-ray (although asthma does not show up on an X-ray).
- RAST (Radio-Allergosorbant Test) measures levels of the allergen antibody IgE against specific antigens. This method is expensive and rarely used in asthma cases. RAST results remain positive for between 6 to 12 months after exposure ceases.
- ELISA (Enzyme Linked Immunosorbant Assay), a similar technique to RAST, is offered by some private clinics.

A WORD OF WARNING

Worries about food allergies in particular and atopic disease generally have led to a rapid increase in the number of private clinics offering to diagnose your allergy, using 'complementary' or 'alternative' methods. Studies suggest that many of these may improve asthma symptoms in some people (see **Chapter 9**).

Some alternative systems, however, rely on monitoring energy or electromagnetic fields. These tests do not come cheap, ranging from £50 to £200 depending on the amount of advice you receive. One method runs an electric current through a clipping of your hair. Another applies an electric impulse to your acupuncture points. Sometimes these programmes are run by people who believe in their effectiveness. In other cases, the practitioners may be cynically preying on people's fears. Most can supply case histories that show they uncovered an allergy missed by conventional medicine.

The majority of GPs do not accept that any of these methods work. Unlike some of the complementary treatments in **Chapter 9**, they usually have not been assessed scientifically. Indeed, physicians regard the explanations behind them as biologically implausible. More seriously, the tests may miss real allergies and diagnose those that do not exist. You should approach these alternative techniques with a healthy degree of cynicism.

CHAPTER 5

ASTHMA TREATMENT

ASTHMA treatment has come a long way since the seventeenth century, when doctors noted that soldiers' asthma improved after they were injured in battle. This improvement probably resulted from a surge in adrenaline, a hormone secreted in response to stress. Adrenaline raises heart rate, pulse rate and blood pressure and also opens the airways, relieving bronchoconstriction.

Doctors in the 1600s consequently tried to treat asthma by deliberately wounding their patients, injecting turpentine into their muscles to produce a sterile abscess. A number of patients, including William III, Prince of Orange, seemed to benefit. As a result, doctors used a variety of substances, including milk, blood and sulphur, to produce sterile abscesses well into the 1930s, despite the dangers involved. Patients treated in this way often developed fevers, and any improvement – probably due to a combination of changes in the immune system and the adrenaline surge – was only short-lived.

Doctors also tried using expectorants and mucolytics to loosen the thick mucus that blocks the lungs of people with asthma. However, expectorants are ineffective and mucolytics can induce bronchoconstriction in sensitive patients. In addition, plant-based treatments were used to open the airways and reverse bronchoconstriction. Some of these relieved patients' symptoms, although they almost always failed to control the underlying inflammation. In fact, the active substances in these herbal remedies worked in a similar way to many of today's bronchodilators.

The double whammy

Today, asthma treatment aims to deliver a 'double whammy'. A **bronchodilator** (also known as a reliever) relieves acute asthma attacks by opening the airways. However, using a bronchodilator alone allows the underlying inflammation in the lungs to rage unchecked – rather like papering over the cracks in your home's walls caused by subsidence: you may not be able to see the cracks for a while, but the subsidence continues unabated and finally your house collapses. If you rely solely on a bronchodilator, you will eventually suffer a worsening of your condition. For more on bronchodilators, see pages 106–121.

As a result, doctors also prescribe an **anti-inflammatory** (also called a preventer), usually a steroid, to control the inflammation (see below). This dual approach to treatment, combined with use of a peak flow meter to detect an increase in inflammation before you develop symptoms, dramatically reduces your likelihood of developing a serious attack. This chapter looks at the benefits and risks of the medicines used to treat asthma, beginning with the foundation of therapy: the anti-inflammatories.

IMPORTANT

All drugs should be used under medical supervision – preferably in adherence with the British Guidelines on Asthma Management (page 137) – and according to a personal management plan agreed with your doctor. See **Chapter 6** for more on management plans.

Steroids

Despite saving the lives of thousands of people with asthma and although they can dramatically improve quality of life, steroids (more correctly called corticosteroids) have a tarnished image. Though they are very effective anti-inflammatories, many people remain reluctant to use even low-dose inhaled steroids. This 'steroid phobia' partly reflects the problem of anabolic steroid abuse, and to some extent the legacy of indiscriminate steroid prescribing in the past. However, their bad reputation is partly justified. Steroid tablets and – to a much lesser extent – inhaled steroids can cause a range of side-effects including osteoporosis, mouth infections and cataracts. So what are steroids and how effective and safe are they?

What are steroids?

Corticosteroids are produced naturally by the adrenal cortex, the outer layer of the adrenal gland, which lies on top of the kidneys. Some steroids secreted from the adrenal cortex – a group known as the glucocorticoids – control the balance of fat, protein and carbo-hydrate in our bodies. Another group – the mineralocorticoids – controls the water and salt balance.

The use of corticosteroids as drugs began in the 1920s, when doctors realised that the symptoms of rheumatoid arthritis cleared up during pregnancy, or when sufferers developed jaundice. However, it was not until the late 1940s that doctors discovered why: corticosteroid production rises during these times. This dampens the inflammation underlying rheumatoid arthritis and thereby alleviates the symptoms. So doctors began treating rheumatoid arthritis with natural corticosteroids, but they did not realise that oral steroids (steroid tablets) can cause serious side-effects and, during the 1950s and 1960s, steroids were prescribed somewhat carelessly. Doctors now recognise that the benefits of steroids come at a price – see 'The risk of side-effects', below.

The image of corticosteroids has also been tainted by anabolic steroid abuse among some athletes, weight lifters and body-builders. Anabolic steroids are chemicals related to testosterone that, abusers believe, increase muscle mass and enhance perfor-mance. However, their performance-boosting benefits are, at best, marginal and the hazards considerable. Anabolic steroids, such as nandrolone and stanozolol, can cause liver damage, depression, sexual problems and a range of other side-effects – although they are occasionally used to treat serious illnesses.

How steroids fight asthma

Steroids are the mainstay of asthma therapy. They are extremely effective at damping down the underlying inflammation of asthma. As inflammation eases, the airways become less sensitive.

Steroids are taken in three ways:

- **inhaled** steroids (including beclomethasone, budesonide and fluticasone) are the commonest way to use steroids in asthma treatment
- **injected** steroids are used to treat acute severe attacks, usually in hospital. Injections do not work more quickly than tablets, but can be used if the patient is unconscious, vomits or is too distressed to swallow
- **tablets**, usually prednisolone, are used to control severe asthma.

The risk of side-effects

Since the 1950s, chemists have developed synthetic corticosteroids with differing potencies that can be applied to the skin, eye or lung, or taken as a tablet to treat a range of inflammatory diseases. These synthetic steroids aim to enhance the efficacy while limiting side-effects. Beclomethasone, budesonide and fluticasone are all synthetic corticosteroids.

The probability that a steroid will cause side-effects depends on the balance between its mineralocorticoid and glucocorticoid actions – most steroids are a mixture of both. Your risk of developing steroid-related side-effects depends on the dose, method of administration and duration of treatment. As a result, the risk of developing side-effects is lower with inhaled steroids than with oral steroids. Similarly, the risk of developing side-effects is higher if you need regular doses of oral prednisolone than if you only need a course once every couple of years.

Adrenal suppression

As we have seen, the adrenal glands secrete natural steroids. The steroids taken by patients to treat inflammatory diseases (such as asthma) suppress production of natural corticosteroids from the adrenal glands. The greater the extent of this 'adrenal suppression', the more likely you are to develop side-effects.

Doctors assess adrenal suppression by measuring levels of the hormone cortisol – low levels suggest that the adrenal gland is functioning poorly. Cortisol secretion fluctuates throughout the day, and a number of external factors – such as stress – also affect cortisol secretion, and test results. Varying susceptibility among individuals and the steroid dose determine a patient's risk of side-effects.

Inhaled steroids

Inhaled steroids, introduced during the 1970s, have transformed the prospects for people with asthma. Used regularly, they reduce the frequency and severity of asthma attacks, and patients need fewer puffs of bronchodilators to treat acute symptoms. However, it takes 10–14 days before symptoms noticeably improve, and the earlier you start steroid treatment, the better. In one study, doctors divided patients into groups according to the length of time they had suffered symptoms of asthma. They then started all the patients on inhaled steroids. Lung function, measured as FEV1 and peak flow (see **Chapter 4**), improved in all the patients. Those whose treatment started within six months of the onset of their symptoms showed the most marked improvement, but patients who had held out for more than two years before beginning inhaled steroids showed the worst outcome, and failed to reach their predicted lung function values. This does not mean that you should not seek help if you have suffered symptoms for many years, as treatment can relieve long-standing asthma; rather, the study underlines the importance of seeking help as soon as possible.

Moreover, if you stop taking inhaled steroids too soon, asthma symptoms and twitchy airways will soon bother you as much as they did before. Symptoms return to pre-treatment values within a week after you stop a six-week course of inhaled steroids, for example. Longer-term treatment, however, has a longer-lasting beneficial effect. Indeed, some doctors hope that asthma might be 'switched off' by long courses of inhaled steroids.

The new inhaled steroids

The first inhaled steroid, **beclomethasone**, was introduced in 1972. This was followed by newer inhaled steroids – **budesonide** and and more recently **fluticasone** – which seem to be at least as effective, and somewhat safer, than beclomethasone.

Table 1: Inhaled steroids currently available

Generic name	Brand(s)
beclomethasone	AeroBec, Beclazone, Becloforte, Becodisks, Becotide, Filair
budesonide	Pulmicort
fluticasone	Flixotide

In one study, 274 people with asthma took either beclomethasone or the same dose of fluticasone for a year.

- 28 per cent of beclomethasone users suffered an acute attack compared to 16 per cent of the fluticasone group.
- 10 per cent of the beclomethasone group endured a severe attack compared to just 2 per cent of those using fluticasone.

Fluticasone is roughly twice as potent as budesonide and beclomethasone, so the British Guidelines on Asthma Management (page 137) suggest that fluticasone be used at half the dose of budesonide or beclomethasone. Most studies confirm that fluticasone and budesonide are at least as effective as beclomethasone at half and the same dose respectively. And as a lower proportion of any swallowed drug enters the bloodstream (see below) fluticasone and budesonide may be less likely to cause side-effects.

The bottom line seems to be that both fluticasone and budesonide are safe and effective. Any difference between them is likely to be marginal. At lower doses there is little to choose between any of the steroids. Beclomethasone seems to be more likely to cause side-effects at higher doses, however. If taking high-dose beclomethasone, you could consider switching to fluticasone or budesonide to reduce the amount of drug that enters your bloodstream, and to lessen the risk of adrenal suppression and side-effects.

It is doubtful whether budesonide has any major advantage over fluticasone, or *vice versa*. Any comparison of the two has to account for the type of inhaler used. A less potent steroid given using a dry powder inhaler (page 127) may be more effective – and better tolerated by the patient – than a more active drug given by a metered dose inhaler without a spacer (page 122), for example.

In other words, it is impossible to separate the effects of the medicine from the effect of the inhaler. Indeed, some experts argue that each combination of 'drug plus delivery system' is unique, so comparisons of different drugs administered using different inhalers cannot be made. Several studies have, however, attempted to evaluate budenoside and fluticasone according to how likely they are to cause adrenal suppression (see below).

The risk of adrenal suppression

- Doses of inhaled steroid below 800mcg daily do not seem to affect adrenal function – or cause side-effects elsewhere in the body.
- About a fifth of patients taking long-term, high-dose (1,500–2,000mcg daily) inhaled steroids show adrenal suppression to an extent that could cause side-effects – see below. However, relatively few patients require such high doses.
- Four studies found that neither budesonide nor fluticasone affect cortisol levels at normal doses, though at higher doses both steroids may slightly reduce adrenal function: budesonide by 10–25 per cent and fluticasone by 6–38 per cent. These falls are within the range of normal values and are unlikely to translate into side-effects.
- Due to fluctuations in cortisol levels due to stress and the time of day, studies comparing adrenal suppression – not surprisingly – show mixed results.

Swallowing inhaled drugs
When you use an inhaler, much of the steroid dose is either swallowed, deposited in your mouth or breathed out. The swallowed portion can be absorbed into the bloodstream in the same way as a tablet. Blood from the gastrointestinal tract (your digestive system) passes through the liver, which acts as the body's waste disposal unit. Here, enzymes break down poisonous chemicals absorbed from food. These enzymes also degrade drugs. Fluticasone is more easily metabolised, or broken down, by these enzymes than budesonide, while budesonide is more susceptible than prednisolone (a steroid tablet), so less fluticasone enters the bloodstream.

Fluticasone and budenoside are therefore less likely to cause side-effects than other steroids that are not so readily metabolised by the body.

The side-effects of inhaled steroids

It is important to remember that, if taken correctly, inhaled steroids cause few, if any, side-effects. At high doses, they may be combined with steroid-sparing drugs that can control symptoms (page 97). Inhaled steroids can be responsible, however, for a variety of side-effects.

- A proportion of inhaled steroid is deposited in the mouth. This reduces local immunity and can trigger an outbreak of thrush (a fungal infection). The yeast responsible, *Candida albicans,* colonises the mouth, causing white spots on the tongue and throat. Oral thrush develops in 5–15 per cent of patients taking inhaled steroids. However, only five per cent or so require treatment. You can reduce the likelihood that you will develop oral thrush by using a spacer and maintaining good oral hygiene (see box below).
- Between a third and a half of all patients develop a hoarse voice, caused by deposits of steroid on the voice box. This condition, called dysphonia, is clearly a particular problem for singers, telephonists and others who use their voice for a living. (It may be less common among people using a dry powder inhaler than those using a metered dose inhaler – see pages 122–9.)
- Inhaled steroids may also cause inflammation of the tongue (glossitis).
- Doses of inhaled steroids over 800mcg daily can cause striae – thin skin that looks like stretch marks.
- A third of people taking 400mcg of budesonide daily bruise easily. Women with asthma are more likely to suffer than men, and the risk seems to increase with age. When the risk of

---

TIP

- Rinsing your mouth immediately after using your inhaled steroid may reduce the risk of dysphonia, glossitis and thrush. But remember to spit rather than swallow: otherwise you will increase the amount of steroid that reaches your gut.

bruising among asthma sufferers taking 800–2,000mcg inhaled budesonide was compared to that among people without asthma, 71 per cent of asthmatics said they bruised easily compared to 32 per cent of those without asthma.

Inhaled steroids and osteoporosis

The jury is still out over whether inhaled steroids undermine bone mass. A fall in bone mass makes it more likely that a person will develop osteoporosis – brittle bone disease – which is a major problem among people taking oral steroids (page 97). People with osteoporosis are vulnerable to disabling fractures of the wrist, hip and spine.

So far, no studies link inhaled steroids with an increased risk of fractures. Nevertheless, some studies using indirect measurements of bone mass, such as the amount of calcium excreted, suggest that high-dose inhaled steroids taken for at least a year may undermine the strength of your skeleton. Studies are further confused by the oral steroids patients took in the past. People who take high-dose oral steroids are also those most likely to require oral prednisolone, which is directly linked with osteoporosis.

INHALED STEROIDS – KEY FACTS

- Inhaled steroids reduce airway inflammation and leave the bronchi less responsive, reducing the frequency and severity of asthma attacks.
- They should be taken regularly, even if you are well.
- Doses of steroids above 800mcg for beclomethasone and budesonide and 400mcg for fluticasone should be administered using a large volume spacer.
- They are generally safe, and certainly far safer than uncontrolled asthma.

Do inhaled steroids impair growth in children?

Whether inhaled steroids undermine childhood growth remains one of the great controversies in asthma – and is often a topic of heated debate at scientific conferences. The controversy is not made any easier to resolve by the fact that asthma itself impairs growth, or that there are problems associated with the methods used to measure growth. For example, some studies into the effects of inhaled steroids on childhood growth use a technique called knemometry – a very sensitive measure able to detect a growth rate of 0.6mm a week in the lower leg. However, short-term knemometry measurements cannot predict a child's final height. Some doctors believe that inhaled steroids may inhibit growth in the short term, but the body compensates and the child 'catches up' in adolescence.

The evidence from numerous studies is mixed. For the prosecution, several studies suggest that inhaled steroids inhibit growth.

- Children with mild asthma aged 7–9 years were treated with beclomethasone (200mcg twice daily) or an inactive placebo. After seven months, children in the steroid group were, on average, 0.95cm shorter than those taking the placebo. The height of the beclomethasone-treated children had not caught up after five months without steroids.
- A year-long study examined 66 children aged 2–8 years who took beclomethasone (200mcg daily) or budesonide (400mcg daily). Over the year, the beclomethasone group showed an average growth rate of 4.3cm while the budesonide group notched up 5.7cm – which is slower than expected.

In the defence of inhaled steroids, different studies point the other way:

- A recent study followed almost 300 children with asthma for up to seven years, comparing their growth and weight to that of children not receiving steroids. In this study, doses of budesonide up to 400mcg daily did not affect growth or weight.
- Another study compared the effects of two different doses of inhaled fluticasone (50mcg or 100mcg) and a placebo on growth in 325 children aged 4–11. Patients discontinued if they required more than two courses of oral steroids or entered puberty. Overall, 261 children completed the year-long study. Results showed that there was no difference in growth between either group.

Overall, it seems that inhaled steroids may *slightly* inhibit growth in *some* children. Any effect is small, however, and will emerge only when a child is prescribed relatively high doses of inhaled steroid. **It is important to remember that uncontrolled asthma is far more likely to undermine a child's growth than steroids.**

TIP

Until researchers resolve the debate, all children taking steroids – at any dose – should have their height regularly measured by the GP or nurse running the asthma clinic. Those needing daily doses of beclomethasone or budesonide over 800mcg, or of fluticasone over 500mcg, should be referred to a paediatrician specialising in asthma until they have finished growing.

Oral steroids

Inhaled steroids are generally effective and safe and most people with asthma are controlled with these alone. However, in some cases – if your asthma proves difficult to control or you suffer a severe worsening of your condition – you may be prescribed a short course of oral steroids (steroid tablets), usually **prednisolone**. Only a very few people with asthma need to take regular courses of oral steroids.

Oral steroids can be life-savers. They are usually given for a few days in children and a week or fortnight among adults to relieve severe, acute asthma. Oral steroids usually suppress the underlying inflammation rapidly, enabling it to be controlled from a day-to-day basis with inhaled steroids. However, the risk of side-effects among oral steroid users is higher than for inhaled steroids. The likelihood of developing side-effects while taking oral steroids depends on the dose and length of treatment.

The risk of adrenal suppression

Long-term oral steroids almost inevitably cause adrenal suppression (page 87). As a result, if your dose is reduced too rapidly you may be left deficient in certain hormones: this can lower blood pressure; cause your asthma to flare up; or, rarely, prove fatal. Doses taken for longer than three weeks are therefore tapered off slowly.

You can take a number of steps to reduce the risk of adrenal suppression, e.g. take oral steroids as a single dose in the morning. Adrenal suppression means you will be less able to cope with the stress of an operation or an infection. The adrenal gland takes up to two years to recover from a course of oral steroids.

TIP

If you take oral steroids for more than a month you should carry a steroid warning card for at least two years after the end of treatment. If you are involved in an accident, for example, you may need to take a higher dose of steroids to overcome adrenal suppression. Tell any health care professional treating you that you take, or have taken, oral steroids.

The effect on the immune system

Oral steroids suppress the immune system, so you are more likely to contract an infection while taking them. In one study, 13 per cent of patients taking oral steroids developed infections compared to eight per cent of those given an inactive placebo. Susceptibility to infection was dose-related: the rate of infection was not any higher among steroid users taking less than 10mg prednisolone a day than in the placebo group.

Even common and generally innocuous infections such as chickenpox can develop into serious problems in people taking oral – and possibly very high-dose inhaled – steroids. If you think you or your child are beginning to develop chickenpox during, or several months after, a course of oral steroids, consult your GP. Signs to watch for are:

- some children and most adults experience malaise, fever, headache and cough before the rash erupts
- a crop of raised spots which develop pus-filled heads and may burst, crust or disappear. This stage lasts for about five days and may be accompanied by a fever
- spots tend to appear on the trunk rather than the limbs.

Apart from increasing the risk that you will contract an infection, oral steroids may mask the signs that usually alert you to your state of health. This means that serious diseases, such as septicaemia and tuberculosis, could be well advanced before you realise that you are ill.

TIP

- Consult your GP if you develop diarrhoea, a fever or vomiting while taking oral steroids.
- Avoid injections of vaccines that induce immunity by producing a mild form of the disease (such as measles or rubella) while taking oral steroids.

The side-effects of oral steroids

You might develop a number of side-effects while taking oral steroids, including those listed below.

Table 2: The side-effects of oral steroids

acne	male impotence
cataracts	muscle weakness, especially in the limbs, shoulder and pelvis
changes in appetite	
changes in fat distribution (typically, fat increases on the face and shoulders – known as 'moon face' and 'buffalo hump')	osteoporosis (especially in post-menopausal women – see below)
childhood growth may be retarded	psychological changes (including agitation, insomnia, depression and euphoria)
children may become excitable	
diabetes	skin thinning (steroids remove protein from the skin, causing stretch marks known as striae)
glaucoma	
increased blood pressure	
increased body and facial hair	skin may bruise easily
indigestion and ulcers	women may find their periods stop

Many of these side-effects are reversible when treatment stops. For example, 'Cushingoid' side-effects – such as moon face, acne and striae – may resolve once treatment stops, as may steroid-induced glaucoma. Similarly, psychological changes abate in nine out of ten cases.

How likely am I to suffer side-effects?

A single, short course of prednisolone (or any other oral steroid) is unlikely to cause serious or permanent side-effects. A typical short course of oral steroids lasts for up to three weeks. Two or three courses of oral steroids a year are relatively safe, especially compared to the dangers of poorly controlled asthma.

Serious side-effects may not emerge at doses of prednisolone below 5mg daily. Above this, the risk increases. Doses below 10mg of prednisolone or its equivalent daily do not usually increase the risk of developing cataracts even when taken for several years – however, three-quarters of people taking 15mg daily for several years develop cataracts. Furthermore, glaucoma develops in up to 40 per cent of patients on long-term steroids and up to 36 per cent of long-term steroid users experience psychological changes, which tend to be more common among patients with a history of mental illness.

Before moving to oral steroids, you could try **steroid-sparing drugs**, which include salmeterol and theophylline. Steroid-sparing drugs are used in conjunction with your inhaled steroid. They allow you to reduce your dose of steroid while maintaining control of your symptoms; or improve symptom control while on the same dose of inhaled steroid. Some patients taking oral steroids develop unacceptable side-effects: steroid-sparing drugs may be prescribed in this case.

TIP

You can take steps to reduce your chance of suffering side-effects:

- take the lowest dose of oral steroids that controls your symptoms for the shortest possible time
- regularly review the risks and benefits of continuing oral steroids with your doctor
- consult your doctor if you think you are suffering unacceptable side-effects.

Oral steroids and osteoporosis

About two million people in the UK suffer from osteoporosis. The disease leaves them vulnerable to debilitating fractures of the wrist, spine and hip, many of which are caused by oral steroids. Despite this, few people taking long-term oral steroids receive treatment to prevent osteoporosis. So why do oral steroids cause osteoporosis? And is there anything you can do to reduce the risk?

Osteoporosis results from the erosion of bone mass in the skeleton as a result of ageing (the leading cause of osteoporosis), oral steroid use or an early menopause. This erosion undermines the skeleton's strength and makes the sufferer prone to fractures. Oral steroids exacerbate an age-related decline in bone mass. We gain some 90–95 per cent of bone mass during adolescence and after peaking during our 20s it declines with age. In men, bone mass declines slowly. But among women, bone mass declines sharply during the 5–10 years following the menopause. After this bone loss then slows, but by this stage much of the structural strength has been lost.

Bone mass declines because the skeleton – despite appearances – is not inert. The stresses and strains of daily life lead to micro-fractures – tiny cracks in the bones. Left unresolved these micro-fractures would undermine the skeleton's strength, so old bone is replaced with new bone throughout life. Depending on the site in the body, 3–25 per cent of the bone mass is replaced each year.

During this 'remodelling', a group of cells known as osteoclasts break down old bone by forming microscopic pits on the bone's surface. Another group of cells – the osteoblasts – fill these pits with new bone, thus healing the micro-fractures. To do this, however, the body needs a continual supply of raw material – calcium and vitamin D. Most of the vitamin D is formed by the action of sunlight on the skin, and from our diet – not everyone gets enough, however – vegans, vegetarians, elderly people and Asian women are especially at risk. Getting enough calcium is more difficult. You would need to drink roughly a litre (two pints) of milk a day to meet your body's requirements, for example. To ensure you get enough of both minerals, take 400–800 iu (10–20 mcg) of vitamin D and 1,000–1,500mg of calcium daily to prevent osteoporosis. The results speak for themselves: in one study of post-menopausal women, those who took supplements containing 1,000mg calcium daily reduced bone loss by up to 67 per cent.

Oral steroids throw the delicate balance of bone remodelling into disarray. During long-term use they reduce bone formation by up to 25 per cent due to three separate factors:

- steroids inhibit the production of new bone
- patients taking oral steroids excrete more calcium in their urine than non-users
- patients taking oral steroids absorb less calcium from food than non-users.

The combination of increased calcium excretion and reduced absorption means that less calcium is available to build new bone. As a result, people with asthma taking long-term oral steroids are much more likely to suffer a fracture – post-menopausal women are especially vulnerable because of the age-related decline in bone mass. For example, 11–42 per cent of people with asthma taking high-dose oral steroids for eight years suffered rib or vertebral (spinal) fractures in one study. Another trial found that just over a third of people with asthma who took an average prednisolone dose of 12mg daily for about nine years experienced a vertebral fracture.

How to reduce side-effects
You can take a number of steps to protect your skeleton from the ravages of oral steroids. These measures will not only reduce your risk of suffering steroid-induced osteoporosis, but will also reduce your likelihood of suffering an age-related fracture:

- take regular weight-bearing exercise (such as rapid walking, jogging and aerobics) for at least 20 minutes three times a week
- avoid smoking
- avoid excessive alcohol consumption
- if you are a post-menopausal woman, consider taking HRT
- ensure your calcium and vitamin D intake is adequate – you may want to consider supplements.

Drugs for steroid-induced osteoporosis
Treatment should begin as soon as possible, although doctors' choice is fairly limited. Bone mass declines most sharply during the first 6–12 months after starting oral steroids, yet the most effective osteoporosis drugs have not been formally approved for use in patients taking oral steroids. In women, the most widely used treatment for post-menopausal osteoporosis is hormone

replacement therapy (HRT), which is not formally approved to reduce steroid-induced bone loss. Some tests found combinations of oestrogen and progestogen (used in HRT) could reduce spinal bone loss in post-menopausal women and those who underwent a hysterectomy while taking long-term oral steroids.

A class of drugs known as the bisphosphonates – which includes etidronate and pamidronate – offers hope to sufferers, though research into their effectiveness still has to be completed. Etidronate and calcium carbonate reduced bone loss in women taking high-dose oral steroids for rheumatoid arthritis, and another study found that pamidronate reduced wrist and spinal bone loss in patients who took long-term steroids for two years. Whether the bisphosphonates affect fracture rates among people taking oral steroids is not known, although studies are underway.

Many specialists advise their patients (and especially women) to take a bisphosphonate or another drug – calcitriol, which is related to vitamin D – to reduce the risk of steroid-induced osteoporosis, though these are not officially approved. Numerous trials are now investigating the treatment and prevention of steroid-induced osteoporosis, and formal approval of some drugs should follow over the next couple of years. Contact the National Osteoporosis Society* for more details.

TIP

- If you take long-term oral steroids, discuss taking bisphospho-nates or calcitriol with your doctor.
- If you have taken several courses of oral steroids, ask your doctor to refer you for a bone scan to determine the extent of any bone loss. A number of treatments are now available for people with confirmed osteoporosis – irrespective of the cause.
- Tell any doctor, dentist, nurse or midwife that you are taking, or have taken, oral steroids.
- If you are a long-term user of oral steroids you could consider wearing a bracelet or necklace with a personal identification number in case you become unconscious. This alerts doctors and other health care professionals to the fact that you suffer from a medical condition. Contact the Medic Alert Foundation* for more information.

Other anti-inflammatories

Nedocromil sodium

Nedocromil sodium (Tilade), which is unrelated to steroids, may be effective in mild asthma. Unlike steroids, which seem to control the entire inflammatory response, nedocromil specifically targets mast cells, preventing them from releasing inflammatory mediators (page 20). In this way nedocromil prevents the nerves in the lung from being irritated (page 22) and is especially effective against cough-variant asthma (page 25) as a result.

Inhaled nedocromil is not as potent as the inhaled steroids – a dose of 4mg puffs of nedocromil four times daily is about as effective as 400mcg beclomethasone twice daily. However, children suffering from asthma-related cough respond to nedocromil within 3–7 days, while inhaled steroids may take several weeks to work. On the whole, more patients respond to steroids – so if your symptoms do not improve after 6–8 weeks your doctor might switch you to inhaled steroids. In some cases, you might use nedocromil if high doses of inhaled steroid do not control your symptoms – this could allow the steroid dose to be reduced by 50–75 per cent.

The benefits of nedocromil

Nedocromil is beneficial for several patients, as the results of an American study show. Doctors studied nedocromil's effects on 1,200 mild-to-moderate asthmatics, aged at least 12 years. The patients took two 4mg puffs of nedocromil four times daily for four weeks.

- Patients' symptoms began to improve after one week and continued to improve for the next three weeks.
- By the end of the study, 82 per cent of patients experienced fewer symptoms.
- Nocturnal asthma and asthmatic cough decreased by almost 50 per cent.

Before treatment, 89 per cent of patients used 'rescue' bronchodilators (page 122). By the end of the study, bronchodilator use declined in 47 per cent. Similarly, the patients' average peak flow was 93 per cent of the predicted value at the start of the study. After one week this increased to an average of 97 per cent, and was nearly 100 per cent by the end of the study. (The impressive peak flow values underline the fact that the patients in this study suffered from mild asthma.)

The risk of side-effects

The only significant side-effects to emerge from the study above were an unpleasant taste (12 per cent of patients) and coughing (8 per cent), similar to the results of other trials.

NEDOCROMIL – KEY FACTS

- Nedocromil is inhaled four times daily, which may cause difficulties for parents who have to trust a teacher or childminder to dose their child. When asthma is well controlled, this may be reduced to twice daily.
- It may help people with mild asthma avoid oral steroids.
- It is particularly suitable for the treatment of asthmatic cough.
- It is especially effective in children, but they must be over six years of age (the drug has not been formally approved for younger children).
- It is very effective in preventing exercise-induced asthma, particularly when taken 20 minutes before working out.
- It is less effective than inhaled steroids.
- Nedocromil comes in a 'mint' flavour that aims to hide the drug's unpleasant taste.

Sodium cromoglycate

Sodium cromoglycate (Cromogen and Intal) was introduced into conventional medicine in 1967. However, sodium cromoglycate was isolated from the seeds of a Middle Eastern plant related to the carrot, *Ammi visnaga*, which was used to treat asthma for centuries. The active ingredient, khellin, was not isolated until 1947. Sodium cromoglycate seems to block the release of inflammatory mediators from mast cells, inhibiting the body's early and late responses in an asthma attack (see **Chapter 1**).

- In inhalation challenge tests (page 79), sodium cromoglycate blocked the bronchoconstriction caused by allergens and non-specific stimuli.
- Regular treatment may prevent an increase in bronchial hyper-reactivity among patients with allergic asthma.

Nevertheless, sodium cromoglycate is a less effective anti-inflammatory than inhaled steroids. If you or your child do not respond well within 4–6 weeks, you should consider switching to inhaled steroids.

The risk of side-effects
Side-effects caused by sodium cromoglycate can include rash, headache and upset stomach, especially among young children with mild asthma, but these are rare.

SODIUM CROMOGLYCATE – KEY FACTS

- Sodium cromoglycate is inhaled four times daily, which may cause difficulties for parents who have to trust a teacher or childminder to dose their child.
- It can be effective in atopic, occupational and exercise-induced asthma.
- In some cases, it prevents – or at least delays – the need for inhaled steroids.
- It is commonly used to treat very young children with asthma.

Zafirlukast

Zafirlukast (Accolate) is the inaugural member of the first new class of anti-inflammatory for asthma to be launched in 20 years. Zafirlukast is relatively safe compared to oral steroids, and is taken twice daily as a tablet, which may improve compliance and could mean that patients do not need to learn how to use an inhaler.

Zafirlukast blocks the action of one class of inflammatory mediators – the leukotrienes. These chemicals, released during the body's immune response, are nearly 10,000 times more potent as a bronchoconstrictor than histamine. Moreover, asthmatics are between 25 and 100 times more sensitive in bronchial provocation tests to one type of leukotriene – leukotriene D4 – than healthy subjects. Zafirlukast specifically targets and blocks the receptor for leukotriene D4, which contributes to bronchoconstriction, inflammation, swelling and mucus secretion. So zafirlukast works differently from the steroids – which are non-selective – and also nedocromil and sodium cromoglycate, which target the mast cell.

The benefits of zafirlukast

Clinical trials show that zafirlukast:

- inhibits the early and late response (**Chapter 1**), preventing bronchoconstriction induced by inhaled histamine for up to six hours
- reduces the need for bronchodilators, improves lung function and symptoms and reduces the number of night-time wakenings
- reduces the number of exacerbations
- works quickly: benefits emerge 1–3 days after starting treatment – somewhat more rapidly than inhaled steroids.

The risk of side-effects

Studies to date suggest that zafirlukast is safe. Side-effects, including headache and gastrointestinal disturbances, tend to be mild. However, some long-term effects may not emerge until thousands of patients have used it safely for several months, or even years. Zafirlukast was not available when the British Guidelines on Asthma Management (page 137) were revised, but it is similar in efficacy to sodium cromoglycate. In Ireland, Finland and the USA, where zafirlukast has been on the market for longer, it is used to treat mild to moderate asthma – roughly step two in the guidelines – in children over 12 years of age. However, the committee that formulates the British Guidelines on Asthma Management believes that more studies comparing zafirlukast to other treatments are needed before they can recommend a position in the programme.

ZAFIRLUKAST – KEY FACTS

- Zafirlukast is a tablet taken twice daily (making it easier to use than inhaled anti-inflammatories).
- It alleviates exercise-induced, atopic and aspirin-induced asthma.
- It is also effective in asthma cases triggered by cold air.
- Benefits may be felt sooner than with inhaled steroids.
- Side-effects are generally mild and transient.
- It has not yet been included in the British Guidelines on Asthma Management.

Ketotifen

Ketotifen (Zaditen) is an anti-inflammatory that may offer some benefit in mild to moderate asthma. However, its cost and relatively high risk of side-effects mean that it is rarely used. Ketotifen acts mainly by blocking the release of histamine during the immune response – see **Chapter 1**. Unlike sodium cromoglycate (which it rivals in effectiveness) ketotifen is taken as a tablet twice a day. If ketotifen does not work within 6–12 weeks, you will probably receive another treatment.

The benefits of ketotifen

Ketotifen reduces the severity of symptoms in 50 per cent of patients after 6 weeks. This rises to 70 per cent after 12 weeks. Lung function tests show little improvement, but do not deteriorate when regular bronchodilators are withdrawn.

The risk of side-effects

Ketotifen causes a number of side-effects, including sedation in between 10 and 20 per cent of older children and adults. Sedation tends to be particularly troublesome during the first two weeks of treatment and then usually wears off. About 1–2 per cent of patients experience dizziness, dry mouth, nausea and headache (which disappear over time), and some gain weight.

The relatively high risk of side-effects means that ketotifen is not widely used. Indeed, the British Guidelines on Asthma Management do not include ketotifen and the National Asthma Campaign★ do not recommend the drug. However, ketotifen may play a role when patients cannot tolerate other drugs or when

---

KETOTIFEN – KEY FACTS

- Ketotifen is a tablet taken twice daily.
- It may be effective for mild to moderate asthma.
- It usually takes six weeks to work.
- It is particularly suitable for patients suffering from more than one allergic disease – asthma, hay fever, eczema and food allergies.
- It is rarely used to treat asthma as side-effects are common.
- If you develop sedation, **do not** drive or operate machinery.

---

asthma, hay fever and eczema are present in the same patient. Similarly, ketotifen can help prevent food allergies when excluding the offending food is either impracticable or nutritionally difficult. You could take ketotifen before, during and for a couple of weeks after a holiday, for example, since this is a time when you are likely to have less control over the content of your food.

Less common drugs

Some anti-inflammatories used to treat arthritis have also been tried in the few asthmatics who are resistant to, or develop severe side-effects to, high-dose oral steroids. For example, **methotrexate** can be prescribed as a steroid-sparing drug when long courses of high-dose oral steroids (over 10mg prednisolone daily) cause unacceptable side-effects – for example, in post-menopausal women suffering from osteoporosis (see 'Oral steroids and osteoporosis', above). This is something of a lottery, however, as some patients show a better response to methotrexate than others – and doctors currently cannot predict who is likely to respond. Moreover, methotrexate's effect can take up to six months to emerge and side-effects – including nausea, blood abnormalities and liver damage – are relatively common. Methotrexate obviously tends to be a drug of last resort.

Gold preparations are widely used to treat rheumatoid arthritis and have been used to treat asthma in Japan for years. A recent study suggested that Auranofin – an oral gold preparation – may help some people suffering from chronic asthma who are not able to cope with oral steroids. However, gold salts are rarely used as they can cause a number of side-effects including rashes and kidney damage.

Bronchodilators

Bronchodilators are almost always used in conjunction with anti-inflammatories. Bronchodilators open the airways, and so can rapidly alleviate acute asthma symptoms. However, bronchodilators do not reduce the underlying inflammation. As a result, it is important to continue taking your anti-inflammatory, even when you feel well. The most widely used bronchodilators are a group of drugs known as 'short-acting beta2-agonists'.

What are short-acting beta2-agonists?

Beta2-agonists, usually called beta-agonists, have been used for more than 30 years in asthma management. They work by artificially stimulating the muscles in the airways to relax and open the airways.

Table 3: Beta2-agonists currently available

Generic name	Brand(s)
fenoterol	Berotec
pirbuterol	Exirel
reproterol	Bronchodil
rimiterol	Pulmadil
salbutamol	Aerolin, Airomir, Asmaven, Maxivent, Salamol, Salbulin, Ventodisks, Ventolin, Volmax
terbutaline	Bricanyl, Monovent
tulobuterol	Respacal

Salbutamol and **terbutaline** are the most widely prescribed beta2-agonists. Usually, patients take inhaled beta2-agonists although a sustained-release tablet containing salbutamol (Volmax) is available. The tablet takes longer to work, though bronchodilation tends to be more sustained than with the inhalers. But the higher likelihood that patients will develop side-effects means that sustained-release salbutamol is not widely used. Bronchodilator syrups may help some children with occasional symptoms, though generally inhalers are less likely to cause side-effects. There are also injectable forms, which may be used in hospital to treat severe attacks. Beta2-agonists can also be used in a nebuliser (page 130).

How beta2-agonists fight asthma

Understanding how beta2-agonists work means making a brief diversion into pharmacology, the science that studies the effects of drugs on the body.

You may remember from biology lessons at school that nerves carry messages to and from the brain. These messages are transmitted along nerves as electrical impulses. When an electrical impulse reaches the end of a nerve it triggers the release of chemical messengers, known as neurotransmitters. These cross a small gap to another nerve or muscle where they lock on to receptors (specialised proteins) on the surface of the nerve, rather like a key fitting into a lock. This switches on a complicated chemical cascade in the nerve or muscle, and the message either continues its journey around the nervous system or contracts or relaxes the muscle.

There are more than 50 chemical messengers, or neurotransmitters, which are made by the body. Many drugs work by binding to receptors (i.e. locking on to proteins on the surface of the nerve) in place of the natural neurotransmitter. In this way they can influence the natural balance of nervous activity.

- **Agonists** bind to the receptor and stimulate the nerve, mimicking the effect of the natural neurotransmitter.
- **Antagonists** (sometimes called 'blockers') bind to the receptor without stimulating it. This prevents the neurotransmitter from binding to the receptor.
- Drugs such as terbutaline (bambuterol) and salbutamol target particular receptors – the beta2-receptors – located in the muscle surrounding the bronchi. These drugs are known as **beta2-agonists**.

The beta2-receptors respond to adrenaline and noradrenaline – natural neurotransmitters that relax the smooth muscle in the airways and increase mucus clearance by encouraging the cilia to beat more rapidly. Drugs that bind to beta2-receptors mimic the action of adrenaline and noradrenaline. As a result, they typically open the airways for 3–6 hours.

The risk of side-effects

In general, inhaled beta2-agonists are safe, although the risk of developing side-effects is greater among people taking oral beta2-agonists.

Remember that beta2-agonists work by binding to receptors known as beta2-receptors? Another type of beta receptor – the beta1-receptor – controls heart function. Beta2-agonists at high doses can bind to beta1-receptors on muscles in the heart. The drug stimulates the heart, so patients may develop cardiovascular side-effects including palpitations, tremor and arrhythmia (abnormal heartbeat). However, it is important to keep the risks in perspective. In a study of over 28,000 people taking either salbutamol or the long-acting beta2-agonist salmeterol (see below):

- 98 people reported palpitations
- 19 reported tachycardia (racing heartbeat)
- 5 reported arrhythmia.

Using beta2-agonists regularly may lead to a decline in lung function – a problem known as **tolerance** or tachyphylaxis. When this
happens, you need to take increasing amounts of the drug to get
the same effect. Beta2-agonists may cause you to develop tolerance
in two ways: first, the body 'adapts' to the high levels of beta2-ago-
nists by 'switching off' beta2-receptors and second, beta2-agonists
reduce the amount of natural anti-inflammatory steroids produced
by the body.

However, several studies suggest that tolerance is unlikely to
develop even if patients take beta2-agonists regularly.

Regular use of beta2-agonists does not offer real benefits and
will not improve either your symptoms or quality of life. You
should therefore use beta2-agonists only to alleviate an acute
attack. For this reason, most specialists do not advocate using the
few combinations of anti-inflammatory and bronchodilator, such
as **Aerocrom** (cromoglycate plus salbutamol) and **Ventide** (salbutamol plus beclomethasone), unless the patient has problems
maintaining a treatment routine, or needs regular doses of both
medicines. Combinations should not be used to alleviate an acute
asthma attack.

How likely am I to suffer side-effects?

- In about one per cent of patients using salbutamol from a
  metered dose inhaler (page 122), the airways narrow when the
  inhaler is used – a problem called **paradoxical bronchoconstriction** (if this happens, you have to wait until the bronchodilation begins to take effect). However, this may be a
  reaction to the propellants in the inhaler rather than the beta2-
  agonist.
- Paradoxical bronchoconstriction may be less likely to happen
  if you use a dry powder inhaler (page 127) – although these
  can trigger coughing in some people.
- Beta2-agonists taken using a nebuliser (page 130) may precipi-
  tate angina and arrhythmia, which could be dangerous among
  some heart disease patients.

Do beta2-agonists increase the risk of dying from asthma?

Some studies suggest that beta2-agonists may increase the risk of dying from asthma *when used without anti-inflammatories*. A Canadian study found that for each canister of beta2-agonist used per month, a patient's risk of death, or near-death due to asthma, roughly triples. Another study confirmed the link between increased risk of death and frequent drug use, but suggested this was the case only if the beta2-agonist was delivered by nebuliser. Regularly using beta2-agonists may increase the amount of allergen reaching the lung. By keeping the airways open, more irritants and allergens penetrate deep into the lung – the very situation that

---

NEW ZEALAND'S ASTHMA EPIDEMIC

Improved asthma management meant that the death rate fell worldwide during the 1980s, yet New Zealand experienced a high level of deaths from asthma between 1976 and 1989 – roughly double the rate in other developed countries. Nothing seemed to explain the increase: the deaths were sudden and unexpected and the usual contributing factors – underestimating the dangers, poor compliance, a delay in seeking help – were not always present.

Doctors now believe that the deaths were due to widespread use of a high-dose beta2-agonist called fenoterol, launched in New Zealand in 1976. The formulation contained a dose of fenoterol some four times higher than the equivalent dose of salbutamol. By 1980, fenoterol had captured 30 per cent of the market – the highest market share in any country.

Eventually, doctors figured out that people with severe asthma using high-dose fenoterol were 13 times more likely to die than those using other bronchodilators. This was because the drug stimulated the beta1-receptors on the heart as well as the beta2-receptors in the lungs, increasing the risk of cardiovascular side-effects – and death.

Consequently, the New Zealand authorities restricted fenoterol's use in 1989 and sales fell. Mortality from asthma declined by two-thirds within a year. Since then, other studies have confirmed that patients taking high-dose fenoterol are more likely to die or suffer a serious attack than those taking salbutamol.

The dose of fenoterol currently available in the UK is lower than that linked to the deaths in New Zealand. When used in accordance with your doctor's instructions, fenoterol is not dangerous.

---

bronchoconstriction evolved to prevent. However, the inflammation provoked by the allergen rages unchecked. This may increase the likelihood that you will develop a severe attack.

Ultimately, the link between beta2-agonists and increased risk of death from asthma is determined by the severity of your symptoms and frequency of drug use, which, of course, are intimately linked. This in turn underlines the importance of taking an anti-inflammatory, since it is only by attacking asthma on both fronts that you will keep your disease under control and lessen the need for beta2-agonists.

A step forward – selective beta2-agonists

Modern beta2-agonists specifically target beta2-receptors in the lung rather than beta1-receptors in the heart, which as we have seen can cause potentially fatal side-effects. Before the New Zealand outbreak, a previous increase in asthma deaths during the 1960s was traced to high doses of an inhaled beta-agonist called isoprenaline (now available as Medihaler-Iso). This bronchodilator targeted both beta1- and beta2-receptors; consequently, high doses were found to increase the risk of death due to cardiovascular side-effects. By contrast, salbutamol pinpoints beta2-receptors 500 times more accurately than it does beta1-receptors. Because of this ability to deliver an effect only where it is needed, modern drugs significantly reduce your likelihood of suffering cardiovascular side-effects.

Long-acting bronchodilators

In general, beta-agonists keep the bronchi open for about 3–6 hours. However, another group of drugs – the long-acting bronchodilators – keep the airways open for up to 24 hours when used twice daily. Long-acting bronchodilators must always be used with an anti-inflammatory but can dramatically improve lung function in a number of patients:

- people with moderate to severe asthma who have frequent symptoms during the day and at night
- people who frequently experience nocturnal symptoms
- people who suffer from exercise-induced asthma.

There are currently two long-acting inhaled bronchodilators on the market: **salmeterol** and **eformoterol**, as well as two tablets: **bambuterol** and sustained-release **theophylline** (see below). If you are prescribed one of these long-acting bronchodilators, make sure you understand the role your drug plays in asthma therapy.

Salmeterol

Salmeterol (Serevent) works in the same way as beta2-agonists – by binding to beta2-receptors (see 'How beta2-agonists fight asthma', above). However, imagine that salmeterol's active part – the part that produces the therapeutic effect – lies at the end of a long chain. The other end of this chain anchors itself to another site deep within the beta2-receptor. Salmeterol's active part 'bounces' in and out of contact with the receptor – like a spring, the chain prevents it moving too far away, so it keeps bumping into the beta2-receptor. The bronchi remain open for 12 hours after a single dose. As a result, to ensure 24-hour effectiveness you take salmeterol twice daily (morning and evening).

Salmeterol may be used as a steroid-sparing drug (page 97) and can be combined with inhaled steroids. In some cases, this may avoid the need to increase the steroid dose. For example, it may be more effective to add salmeterol to beclomethasone than to double the steroid dose – in terms of both lung function and symptom relief – and may enable you to avoid oral steroids. The British Guidelines on Asthma Management suggest that the role of combining a long-acting bronchodilator and inhaled steroids needs further research. It is, however, worth asking your doctor about trying salmeterol before increasing your steroid dose.

The benefits of salmeterol
Salmeterol can dramatically improve the symptoms of asthma.

- In two studies involving more than 500 patients suffering from mild to moderate asthma, morning and evening peak flows were higher among salmeterol users than those taking regular salbutamol.
- Patients taking salmeterol experienced fewer and less severe day- and night-time symptoms and used fewer doses of inhaled rescue bronchodilator.
- The number of nights during which patients were disturbed

by asthma fell by 52 per cent, compared to a 21 per cent decline among patients using a placebo.

The risk of side-effects

Side-effects .you might experience are those common to other beta2-agonists, such as tremor, increased heart rate and palpitations. These side-effects are usually minor and decline during regular use. It was thought at first by some doctors that keeping the bronchi open might lead to the lungs being overloaded with allergens, which could increase the risk of an attack. Reassuringly, studies to date suggest that salmeterol does *not* lead to an increase in attacks, provided you regularly take an anti-inflammatory. Moreover, salmeterol does not appear to be any more likely to induce tolerance (page 109) than short-acting bronchodilators.

There are some cautionary points, however. Although salmeterol is licensed for use in people with asthma over the age of four years, its long-term effects in children are not known and among those who take it, the drug has to be used carefully. Moreover, the importance of using anti-inflammatories in addition was revealed by a study performed soon after its launch. In this study, 25,000 people with moderate to severe asthma received either salbutamol or salmeterol. Twice as many people received salmeterol as salbutamol. However, 12 people taking salmeterol died compared to two in the salbutamol group. Studies of death rates among people with asthma suggest that this should have been ten in the salmeterol group and five in the salbutamol group.

There are several explanations for the increased number of deaths among the salmeterol group. First, the difference could be due to chance – after all, the number of excess deaths was just two patients out of 25,000. Second, the results of the study were presented in 1992. Since then, doctors have become more aware of the need for adequate anti-inflammatory medications, especially among patients taking long-acting bronchodilators. Third, patients may have used the drugs incorrectly. Salmeterol is a powerful drug and can dramatically improve symptoms – as a result, patients may have deliberately or subconsciously reduced the dose of anti-inflammatory.

How likely am I to suffer side-effects?

Salmeterol given by a metered dose inhaler is especially likely to cause paradoxical bronchoconstriction (page 109). This is probably triggered by the propellants in the inhaler, which make the bronchi constrict before the drug has a chance to take effect – salmeterol takes a while to begin to work.

Using salmeterol safely

Since 1992, when the results of the study above were published, many thousands of patients have received salmeterol. The medicine is now an established and useful part of asthma management and generally regarded as safe. Indeed, a later, similarly sized study to that performed just after its launch reported that fewer patients died while taking salmeterol than expected. Nevertheless, you should follow some simple rules in order to use salmeterol (and eformoterol, see below) safely.

- **Do not use salmeterol to alleviate an acute attack**. Use short-acting inhaled beta2-agonists instead. Salmeterol can take 20 minutes to exert its maximum effect, compared with between four and ten minutes for salbutamol, so salmeterol is relatively ineffective in acute asthma; indeed, about 20 people worldwide may have died as a result of taking salmeterol for an acute attack. Always carry your short-acting bronchodilator in case you need to use 'rescue' medication (page 122).

- **Do not use salmeterol more than twice daily**. The body eliminates salmeterol more slowly than short-acting inhaled beta2-agonists, so following excessive use of the drug blood levels of salmeterol can rise, leading to side-effects. (Side-effects are rarely a problem if you take salmeterol twice daily.)

SALMETEROL – KEY FACTS

- Salmeterol is a long-acting inhaled bronchodilator taken twice daily.
- It may be particularly effective combined with inhaled steroids (200–2,000mcg for beclomethasone or budesonide, or 100–1,000 mcg for fluticasone) and could reduce the need for oral steroids.
- It alleviates nocturnal asthma.
- It is more likely to cause paradoxical bronchoconstriction than short-acting beta2-agonists (pages 107–9).
- It may cause cardiovascular side-effects in some cases.
- While it is licensed for use in children over four years, the effects of long-term use in children are not known.

- **Do not discontinue anti-inflammatory therapy** even if you feel well. Doing so could provoke a serious, even fatal, attack.

Eformoterol

Eformoterol (Foradil) works in a different way from salmeterol. Rather than 'bouncing' in and out of contact with the beta2-receptors, eformoterol binds strongly to the receptors and is absorbed by the fatty membrane surrounding each cell. When levels in the blood fall, eformoterol slowly leaches out of the fat like a reservoir to top them up. This results in a longer duration of action.

The benefits of eformoterol
Fewer studies have been performed on eformoterol, but its side-effects and effectiveness seem to be roughly similar to those of salmeterol. For example, improvements in lung function, nocturnal symptoms and reduced use of 'rescue' bronchodilators appear to be similar to those produced by salmeterol (see 'The benefits of salmeterol', above). Eformoterol acts more rapidly than salmeterol. But like salmeterol, eformoterol is **not** appropriate as a 'rescue' bronchodilator (page 122).

The risk of side-effects
There is no evidence that eformoterol increases the risk of a severe asthma attack or induces tolerance.

Overall, there seems to be little to choose between eformoterol and salmeterol in terms of either effectiveness or side-effects. However, whereas children over the age of four can use salmeterol, only adults over 18 should use eformoterol. **The rules for using salmeterol safely (see above) also apply to eformoterol. Read this section carefully.**

EFORMOTEROL – KEY FACTS
- Eformoterol is a long-acting bronchodilator taken twice daily.
- It is licensed for use only in adults over the age of 18.
- It should not be used to relieve an acute asthma attack.
- Side-effects and benefits are similar to those with salmeterol (see above).

Bambuterol

Bambuterol (Bambec) is a tablet that is broken down by the body to release an active ingredient: the long-acting beta2-agonist **terbutaline**. However, oral beta2-agonists are more likely than inhaled drugs to provoke side-effects including tremor, headache and dizziness.

Few direct comparisons with other drugs have been made, but in studies into nocturnal asthma, salmeterol (page 112) seems more likely to reduce the number of nocturnal wakings than bambuterol. Bambuterol should therefore be prescribed only if both salmeterol and eformoterol fail to control symptoms adequately.

BAMBUTEROL – KEY FACTS

- Bambuterol is a sustained-release tablet taken once daily.
- It can be useful if inhaled bronchodilators fail to control symptoms.
- It is more likely to cause side-effects than inhaled beta2-agonists.

Theophylline

Theophylline is a member of a naturally occurring family of plant-derived chemicals – the xanthines – which also contains caffeine and theobromine. Indeed, you probably drink theophylline every day: tea contains small amounts. Xanthines, such as theophylline, relax the ring of muscle surrounding the bronchi. This is why a strong cup of coffee may be able to stave off a very mild asthma attack (though this is not recommended long-term as a treatment). Theophylline also improves the mobility of bronchial mucus, unblocking the airways.

Theophylline, which is taken orally, has been used since 1922, and is available as a number of brands (see table below). More recently, theophylline was joined by the related drugs amino-phylline and choline theophyllinate. Theophylline is given as a sustained-release tablet, meaning that the active ingredient is slowly released into the gut, keeping the bronchi open for up to 12 hours.

Table 4: Theophylline preparations currently available

Generic name	Brand(s)
theophylline	Lasma, Nuelin, Slo-Phyllin, Theo-Dur, Uniphyllin Continus
aminophylline	Pecram, Phyllocontin Continus
choline theophyllinate	Choledyl

The benefits of theophylline

For many years, theophylline was a drug on the wane – but it now seems poised to make a comeback. Doctors re-evaluated theophylline following the research that suggested it is anti-inflammatory as well as a bronchodilator – it seems to inhibit the T lymphocyte, a type of white blood cell involved in asthma (page 18). Importantly, the anti-inflammatory effects emerge at doses below those that cause bronchodilation – as a result, anti-inflammatory doses are below those that may lead to side-effects.

However, theophylline is not a particularly powerful anti-inflammatory. Tests on animals suggest that theophylline is about as potent as sodium cromoglycate, and in studies comparing theophylline and inhaled steroids, the steroids tend to perform better. In one study of children with moderately severe asthma, those taking theophylline were more likely to suffer side-effects – including headache, tremor, nausea and vomiting – than those using inhaled beclomethasone. Children taking beclomethasone were less likely to need rescue bronchodilators or oral steroids than those taking theophylline.

Comparisons with inhaled bronchodilators suggest that salmeterol produces a greater improvement in morning and evening peak flow, and controls daytime symptoms better, while theophylline tends to have a longer duration of action and can prevent nocturnal asthma. Nevertheless, direct comparisons suggest that theophylline is worse at controlling symptoms and causes more side-effects. However, combining inhaled steroids and oral theophylline is more effective than either drug used alone.

For example, 56 children started using theophylline. Of the 16 children using oral steroids in this group, 15 were able to stop taking them, while 33 children in the same study reduced their inhaled dose and ten stopped taking steroids altogether.

In a recent study, theophylline was withdrawn from the regimens of 25 patients with severe asthma. Their condition and lung function deteriorated markedly despite receiving a high average dose (1,548mcg daily) of inhaled steroid.

The fact that these patients deteriorated despite high-dose inhaled steroids suggests that theophylline works by a different mechanism to steroids. This is why some doctors believe that patients may benefit from theophylline prescribed as a steroid-sparing drug (page 97) to prevent them moving from low- to high-dose steroids. If low-dose theophylline has a future in asthma management, it is therefore most likely to be used as an addition to inhaled steroids, as outlined in steps three and four of the British Guidelines on Asthma Management (page 138). Some researchers hope that theophylline might be repositioned to step two, though the British Guidelines on Asthma Management suggest that further studies are needed before this can be recommended.

The risk of side-effects

Over the years, side-effects have traditionally proved theophylline's Achilles heel. The problem with theophylline is that the blood levels which open the airways are roughly half those that cause side-effects. So the theophylline dose must be carefully tailored to the patient's response – the patient takes increasing amounts of theophylline until either the asthma is controlled or side-effects emerge. To ensure levels remain within safe limits, patients taking theophylline often need frequent blood tests.

Side-effects (see box) are less of an issue with lower anti-inflammatory doses. Used as a bronchodilator, however, theophylline tends to cause a number of unpleasant side-effects – similar to those you might feel if you drink too much caffeine. Moreover, many external factors influence the way the body metabolises (breaks down) theophylline, which can make theophylline ineffective or produce unacceptable side-effects. Smoking and alcohol, for example, lower blood levels – which may make theophylline ineffective as a bronchodilator. Similarly, viral infections, heart failure and liver disease can raise blood levels – sometimes into the toxic range – and a wide range of drugs can affect xanthine levels. Because of this, you should check with your doctor or pharmacist about drug interactions.

THEOPHYLLINE'S SIDE-EFFECTS

abdominal pain, diarrhoea, headache, heart disturbances, insomnia, nausea, nervousness, tremor, vomiting.

Side-effects are relatively common, for example about a third of children taking theophylline experience stomach upsets, sleep disturbances and behavioural changes. The latter attract concern from parents and doctors, although some of these behavioural changes may be in the mind of the beholder. Tests show over-anxious parents may exaggerate perceived alterations in their child.

One trial studied 8- to 12-year-old children whose parents claimed they suffered from impulsiveness, hyperactivity, altered mood and impaired attention while taking theophylline. Researchers measured attention, impulsiveness, memory, activity level and mood. The children showed a mild increase in anxiety and tremor of the dominant hand, but made fewer attention errors than the parents thought.

As a result of problems with side-effects, physicians in the UK regard theophylline as a second-line drug, suitable to be prescribed only in cases where other drug combinations do not work. British treatment guidelines do not recomment its use until step three of the management plan (page 138).

THEOPHYLLINE – KEY FACTS

- Theophylline is a long-acting bronchodilator usually taken as a sustained-release tablet once daily.
- It acts as a bronchodilator and probably as a mild anti-inflammatory.
- It can be effective in combination with inhaled steroids and may delay the need for high doses of steroids.
- It can be useful in the treatment of children with severe asthma.
- It carries a high risk of side-effects.
- You may need regular blood tests.
- **If you take theophylline and are prescribed another drug or buy one from a chemist, check with your doctor or pharmacist that there will be no interaction.**

Anticholinergics

Anticholinergics are usually prescribed when high-dose inhaled steroids combined with salmeterol fail to control a patient's symptoms adequately. Two inhaled anticholinergics – **ipratropium bromide** and **oxitropium bromide** – are currently available.

Table 5: Anticholinergics currently available

Generic name	Brand(s)
oxitropium bromide	Oxivent
ipratropium bromide	Atrovent, Steri-Neb
ipratropium with salbutamol	Combivent
ipratropium with fenoterol	Duovent

How do anticholinergics fight asthma?

As described earlier (page 108), drugs work by either blocking or stimulating receptors on nerves and muscles. Every muscle and organ is supplied with at least two opposing nerves – one to cause contraction, the other to cause relaxation. The ring of muscle surrounding the bronchi is supplied with nerves that release noradrenaline, a neurotransmitter which stimulates the muscles and opens the airways – beta2-agonists mimic noradrenaline. The muscle surrounding the bronchi is also supplied with nerves that release a neurotransmitter called acetylcholine, which binds to a different class of receptor. This contracts the bronchi and closes the airways. Anticholinergics bind to 'cholinergic' receptors in the bronchi, but instead of stimulating the nerves they block the receptors, preventing acetylcholine from binding there. As a result, anticholinergics keep the airways open. The maximum effects of ipratropium and oxitroprium tend to emerge relatively slowly, but altogether the former keeps the bronchi open for up to eight hours and the latter for about 12 hours.

Some studies suggest that the anticholinergics may be particularly effective in the treatment of older people suffering from COPD (Chronic Obstructive Pulmonary Disease – page 65). Ipratropium is available in combination with the beta2-agonists salbutamol and fenoterol (see Table 5). In people with COPD, this combination may produce a more profound bronchodilation than either salbutamol or ipratropium alone. However, in asthma combinations tend to be used only when compliance (page 59) is poor.

In a 12-week study of 534 patients with an average age of 63, a combination of salbutamol and ipratropium improved FEV1 by 31–33 per cent – compared with figures of 24–25 per cent for ipratropium alone and 24–27 per cent for salbutamol. There was no increase in the number of side-effects among patients taking the combination of salbutamol and ipratropium.

The risk of side-effects

Side-effects are rare. But patients suffering from glaucoma and benign prostatic hyperplasia should use anticholinergics with caution, especially if taken by a nebuliser (page 130). If you are taking nebulised anticholinergics, be sure to use a mouthpiece.

- **Glaucoma** is caused by an increase in pressure inside the eye. This damages the delicate layer of nerves – the retina – that transmits light into the brain, where it is translated into vision. Patients with acute glaucoma, especially those who do not use nebulisers with a mouthpiece, may find anticholinergics increase the pressure in the eye, thereby speeding the destruction of the retina. The risk is increased among those combining nebulised salbutamol and ipratropium.
- **Benign prostatic hyperplasia** is a non-cancerous enlargement of the prostate gland in men, which lies at the base of the bladder surrounding the urethra (the tube urine passes through). This enlargement causes a variety of urinary symptoms, including incontinence. In men with benign prostatic hyperplasia, anticholinergics can trigger a worsening of symptoms and perhaps the inability to pass urine.

Inhaler devices

A wide range of anti-inflammatories and bronchodilators are available to treat asthma, and as we will see in **Chapter 10** these are being joined by a number of newer agents. However, the safety and effectiveness of the drugs themselves are not the end of the story. To be most effective, the medicine needs to reach the lung. This is not a problem with oral drugs, which are transported to the lung by the blood. However, most patients inhale asthma treatment. Your choice of inhaler device can markedly influence the effectiveness of treatment and the risk that you will develop side-effects.

There are several types of inhaler device on the market. These fall into three main groups:

- **metered dose inhalers**
- **dry powder inhalers**
- **breath-actuated devices.**

While the number of inhalers appears confusing, at least this means you can work with your doctor or nurse to individualise treatment. If you find one inhaler difficult to use, ask your doctor to prescribe an alternative. Although the output of different steroid inhalers can vary by 36 per cent, this is relatively unimportant. After all, up to half of people with asthma do not comply with treatment (follow medical guidelines correctly). The key is to **find an inhaler you are comfortable with – and use it!**

IMPORTANT

Even for people who do not use bronchodilators often, it is essential to keep a spare **'rescue' bronchodilator** to hand in case you suffer an unexpected asthma attack, or run out of medication. Ideally, you should keep the extra inhaler with you, or at least where it will be accessible at school or work. If you have been taking your drugs correctly, monitoring your peak flow and following a self-management plan, an attack out of the blue is likely to be rare.

Metered dose inhalers

Pressured metered dose inhalers (MDIs) – sometimes known as 'puffers' – are the commonest way to deliver drugs for asthma. Worldwide, 70 per cent of people with asthma rely on MDIs for their medication. However, there are two main problems with MDIs.

First, although patients usually shake the inhaler to see if they are running out of medication, MDIs contain enough propellant (the gas that carries the active drug and makes the sound) and drug for about 30 more actuations (pressing actions) than the number of doses of drug in the inhaler. As a result, it is possible to inhale nothing but propellant when you reach the end of a canister – you cannot tell from the sound that the propellant no longer contains the drug. Obviously, this means that patients are more likely to suffer an asthma attack.

In one study, doctors interviewed 51 patients aged 13–22:

- 37 people waited until their inhaler was empty before replacing it
- 36 sometimes ran out of inhaler
- 33 people reported becoming wheezy
- only 15 always carried their inhaler
- 19 had no spare inhaler.

These findings highlight the importance of always keeping a spare bronchodilator close by.

The second problem is that only 50 per cent of people use MDIs correctly. The aerosol spray containing the drug exits the inhaler at 15 metres per second – that's 75 miles per hour. This means that once you press the inhaler, you have just 0.1–0.2 seconds to inhale. Not surprisingly, timing faults are the commonest error in inhaler technique among people using MDIs. Poor co-ordination means that less drug reaches the lungs and more is deposited in the mouth and throat. This increases the risk of side-effects from steroids and reduces the effectiveness of both anti-inflammatories and bronchodilators. Even in people with good inhaler technique, 80 per cent of the inhaled dose from an MDI may remain in the mouth and throat.

A number of other common faults reduce the amount of drug reaching the lung:

- stopping inhaling when the cold jet of propellant hits the back of the throat (doctors describe this as the 'cold Freon' effect)
- actuating (pressing) the inhaler too early or too late – before or after breathing in
- pressing the canister twice during the same breath
- not placing the mouthpiece correctly in the mouth
- puffing out the cheeks (which traps the drug in the corner of the mouth).

See the box opposite for how to use an MDI the right way.

HOW TO USE AN MDI CORRECTLY

- Remove the mouthpiece cover and check that the mouthpiece is clean and clear of any obstruction. If you leave an inhaler in your pocket without the cover, fluff and even coins can become caught in the mouthpiece.
- Shake the inhaler well. The drug particles 'float' on the propellant. Shaking the MDI ensures that each actuation delivers an equal amount of drug.
- Cold canisters can reduce the amount of drug delivered from an MDI, so on cold days warm the inhaler in your hands. However, do not dismantle the MDI or place it on a heater or radiator.
- Breathe out as far as you can and place your lips around the mouthpiece. Leaving your mouth open can lead to the drug being deposited on the lips, face and teeth.
- Breathe in steadily and press – 'actuate' – the device. Breathing in slowly and steadily reduces turbulence in the upper airways, so more drug reaches the lower airways.
- Hold your breath for ten seconds, if possible. Holding your breath increases the amount of small particles deposited on the airway walls.
- If you need more than one puff, wait a minute before beginning again. Always shake the canister between doses.
- Replace the mouthpiece cover.

Spacers

The various types of spacers reduce the amount of drug deposited in the mouth, increase the proportion reaching the lung and overcome the 'cold Freon' effect. As less steroid remains in the mouth and more reaches the lung, the risk of local side-effects, such as thrush, is less than with MDIs used alone. Moreover, as there is less in the mouth to swallow, the risk of other side-effects may also be less. If you use an MDI, steroid doses of above 800mcg of beclomethasone and budesonide and 400mcg of fluticasone should be administered using a large volume spacer.

The simplest spacer is a tube that slows the spray of medication. **Large volume spacers**, also called chamber devices, come in two clear plastic sections that you clip together. A valve at one end of the spacer opens only when you breathe in and shuts when you breathe out. In this way, large volume spacers hold the drug particles in suspension until you inhale them. As a result, there is no need to co-ordinate actuation and inhalation. However, large volume spacers are unwieldy and do not fit easily into a bag or pocket. This makes taking asthma drugs more obvious, especially in social situations. Teenagers, especially, may feel that the large volume spacer draws attention to their asthma.

However, large volume spacers increase the amount of drug deposited in the lung.

- In one study of people using an MDI alone, nine per cent of the drug reached the lung and 81 per cent was deposited in the mouth and throat. The remainder was either left in the MDI or exhaled.
- With the large volume spacer (in this case the Nebuhaler), the amount of drug reaching the lung increased to 15–20 per cent, with just 11–17 per cent deposited in the mouth and throat. About 56–68 per cent remained in the chamber, depending on the number of actuations.

Tube spacers aim to strike a balance between portability and the benefits of the larger spacers. A short tube is attached to the end of the inhaler, which allows the propellant to evaporate. This reduces the 'cold Freon' effect and slows the particles, which increases the amount of drug that reaches the lung. However, some co-ordination is still needed to use the device and tube spacers are unsuitable for children under five.

The **AeroChamber** is a small and compact tube spacer. It contains a valve that 'whistles' if you inhale too quickly. Another advantage is that the AeroChamber is replaced only once a year. Some MDIs now have an integral spacer – these are easier to use than a separate spacer and traditional MDI. The **Babyhaler** (currently not available on prescription) may be a good alternative for young children. It is half the size of adult spacers and is used with a silicon mask – parents can easily learn how to operate it (see 'The three ages of asthma', page 156). In an emergency, you could take a large disposable coffee cup and cut a hole in the bottom of a size that snugly fits the inhaler mouthpiece. The open end of the cup can then be placed over the baby's face – rather like a mask – and the inhaler actuated through the hole.

See the box below for information on using a spacer the right way.

HOW TO USE A SPACER CORRECTLY

- Shake the MDI.
- Fit the MDI into a hole at the other end of the spacer.
- Press the inhaler.
- Breathe in slowly and steadily through the mouthpiece in one breath. Unlike using an MDI alone, you do not have to time this exactly and can breathe in for up to ten seconds (the sooner the better, though).
- If you feel breathless, breathe as comfortably as possible.
- Actuate the inhaler again when you need to.
- Hold your breath for 5–10 seconds. If you are unable to hold your breath, you can take shallow 'tidal' breaths in and out half a dozen times.

You may need to service your spacer once a week. Wash it in warm water and mild detergent, rinse it and leave it to dry. Do not wipe it dry – this can lead to a build-up of static electricity, so particles of drug are more likely to stick to the inside and less reaches your lung. It is worth washing a new spacer before you use it for the first time, to discharge any static electricity left over from the manufacturing process. You should replace a large volume spacer every six months or so.

Which device fits which drug?

Inhalers and spacers come in various shapes and sizes. Manufacturers make spacers to fit their own brand of MDI. So you need to use the correct inhaler and spacer.

Table 6: Some spacer – inhaler combinations

Spacer	Inhaler
Nebuhaler	Bricanyl (bronchodilator), Pulmicort (steroid)
Volumatic	Serevent, Ventolin (bronchodilator), Becotide, Becloforte, Flixotide (steroids), Cromogen (sodium cromoglycate)
Fisonair	Intal (sodium cromoglycate)
AeroChamber	Fits all inhalers in baby, child and adult sizes with a mask

Dry powder inhalers and breath-actuated devices

Dry powder inhalers (DPIs) – for example Accuhaler, Diskhaler, Easi-Breathe, Rotahaler, Turbohaler – and breath-actuated devices, such as the Autohaler, are triggered when you inhale and are available containing a variety of bronchodilators and anti-inflammatories.

However, the main difference between DPIs and MDIs is that you do not have to actuate the inhaler, which reduces the need for co-ordination and manual dexterity. There are differences between the various inhalers, so make sure you understand how to use yours and ask for the information leaflet provided by the manufacturer.

DPI and breath-actuated devices increase the amount of drug deposited in the lung. Indeed, steroid doses delivered by the Turbohaler may be halved compared to those from the MDI. DPI and breath-actuated devices generally produce a greater increase in peak flow, patients may need fewer doses of 'rescue' medication compared to MDIs and they are less likely to suffer a worsening of their condition.

- An MDI deposits about eight per cent of a dose of terbutaline (page 00) in the lung. The Turbohaler (a DPI) increases the amount of drug deposited to about 20 per cent.
- Many patients prefer the newer devices. In one study, 56 per cent preferred the Turbohaler to an MDI. Just 26 per cent preferred the MDI. The remainder expressed no preference.

However, DPIs and breath-actuated devices still need a certain amount of manual dexterity to be used correctly. Moreover, individual devices have advantages and disadvantages.

- **Accuhaler** was launched in 1995, is relatively easy to use and contains 60 doses – roughly a month's supply. A counter tells you how many doses remain.
- **Autohaler** is primed by lifting a lever. This may be difficult for people with weak wrists or arthritis. The device clicks when you breathe in: this sound and the 'cold Freon' effect (page 123) can stop people inhaling. Care has to be taken to avoid blocking air vents on inhalation; nevertheless, elderly people with poor inhaler technique find the Autohaler easier to use than an MDI or Rotahaler. Moreover, the Autohaler may triple the amount of drug deposited in the lung among

people with poor inhaler technique. Though the Autohaler does not offer any additional benefits for people who already have good inhaler technique, it is less obtrusive than an MDI and spacer, and most patients find the Autohaler easier to use than this conventional combination.

- **Cyclohaler** *see* **Spinhaler**.
- **Diskhaler** must be loaded with a disk that contains eight doses of drug. Loading the disk, which comes with the inhaler, requires good sight and manual dexterity and you need to apply firm pressure to burst the 'blister' that contains the drug. Schoolchildren can use this device successfully. The Diskhaler requires regular maintenance, which mainly consists of brushing the components, and will probably need to be replaced after three months.
- **Easi-Breathe** is a breath-actuated inhaler with an integral spacer. It is easier to use than the Autohaler, and won the 1997 Prince Charles Innovative Design Award. Currently, it is available with salbutamol and beclomethasone.
- **Rotahaler** uses a capsule – known as a Rotacap – which must be loaded correctly. This is straightforward, though people with poor manual dexterity as well as the blind and partially sighted may experience problems. You can load only one dose at a time, which could be a problem during an asthma attack – unless your doctor supplies several inhalers, you cannot pre-load several doses. Rotacaps need to be protected from damp.
- **Spinhaler** and **Cyclohaler** are similar to the Rotahaler. They also have the same main limitation: i.e. both must be loaded before each inhalation.
- **Turbohaler** must be held upright during use. Some patients with weak or painful hands may find turning the dose-release grip difficult, although an additional hand grip – the Turboaid – is available to facilitate use. Plus points are that the Turbohaler does not need repeated loading and has been designed to indicate when it is almost empty.

On the downside, DPIs and breath-actuated inhalers cannot be used with a spacer. In addition, the speed at which you inhale influences the amount of drug deposited in the lung. For example, at a 'normal' flow rate, 28 per cent of a dose of budesonide from a Turbohaler is deposited in the lung, while among people who inhale at a slower rate this falls to 15 per cent. Output (and, there-fore, deposition) from the Accuhaler seems to be constant across a wide range of respiratory flows.

The advantages of DPIs and breath-actuated inhalers seem clear. However, while cost-containment in the National Health Service remains of overriding importance, MDIs offer one critical advan-tage: they are cheap – one reason why they remain widely pre-scribed. If you are not happy with your MDI, see below for suggestions on how to ask your doctor about switching inhalers.

TIP

If you currently use an MDI with a spacer but think there is a case for trying a DPI, you could take the following approach.

- If you are having difficulties with the current set-up, point out that you find using and transporting a large volume spacer difficult in the office, classroom, lecture hall or wherever, and in social situations. (This could be counter-productive if it sug-gests to your doctor that you are developing a bad track record when it comes to following the prescribed treatment.)
- Alternatively, you might want to propose a compromise. You should need to take your steroid only twice a day, so ask your doctor if you can use a spacer and an MDI for steroids at home, provided you can have a less obtrusive breath-actuated inhaler or DPI to carry around with you for your bronchodilator.

New inhalers: protecting your lungs and the ozone layer

At present MDIs, the Autohaler and the Easibreath are propelled with chlorofluorocarbons (CFCs). Although CFCs are harmless to the lung, when released into the atmosphere they damage the hole in the ozone layer. This allows more harmful ultra-violet (UV) light to penetrate to earth. The CFCs in one inhaler could destroy up to a ton of ozone. As a result, CFCs are being phased out and it is likely that the CFCs used as propellants in MDIs will be phased out altogether over the next few years. The first CFC-free inhaler – the **Airomir**, containing salbutamol – was introduced in 1996 and others will follow.

The new non-CFC propellants underwent extensive safety tests. Indeed, the testing was more extensive than that originally carried out on CFC propellants. CFC-free inhalers are safe, but you may experience some changes when switching to the new version. The 'flavour' of the new propellant as well as the sensation of the propellant in the mouth differs from existing inhalers. The inhaler may also be a different shape, feel and weight. Nevertheless, patients consider the inhalers containing the new propellant to be just as acceptable as the CFC version. In fact, in one test about 63 per cent preferred the new inhaler, while only 11 per cent preferred the CFC version. About 98 per cent were able to switch inhalers easily.

Changing over may affect your drug dose. With the exception of salbutamol, which is the same in CFC-free inhalers as in older inhalers, your dose of inhaled steroids or other drugs may alter when switching to a new inhaler. Changing a tried-and-trusted inhaler is always stressful, but it is important to remember that the new versions are as effective and safe as your existing medicine. Nevertheless, it is prudent to monitor your symptoms and peak flow (page 72) during the switch.

TIP

You should be able to recognise the difference between anti-inflammatories (preventers) and bronchodilators (relievers). To help you, asthma inhalers are colour-coded.

- Anti-inflammatories (e.g. inhaled steroids) are usually brown, but may also be red, orange or yellow.
- Bronchodilators (including beta2-agonists) are usually blue.

Nebulisers

Nebulisers allow patients to inhale large amounts of drug with little effort. They are used either in emergencies under medical supervision, or to treat people with severe asthma. Nebulisers are devices about the size of a small briefcase, which use ultrasound or compressed air or oxygen to force drug solutions through a narrow hole. This creates a fine mist of tiny droplets, which the patient inhales through a face mask or mouthpiece. The small size of the droplets enables them to penetrate deep into the lung. Nebulisers can be used by patients of all ages to administer a wide range of drugs, including bronchodilators (e.g. salbutamol and terbutaline), anticholinergics (ipratropium) and anti-inflammatories (sodium cromoglycate and budesonide).

NEBULISERS – KEY FACTS

- Large volume spacers are often just as effective as a nebuliser, and in an emergency can be used to deliver the same dose of bronchodilator. Make sure you really cannot use one of the many inhalers available before buying a nebuliser.
- Nebulisers are not usually available on the NHS. Some hospitals and pharmaceutical companies may provide them on loan. Some charities help patients purchase nebulisers. People on a low income should contact the local Citizens Advice Bureau (listed in your phone book) to see if local funds are available.
- Nebulisers can be bought VAT-free on a doctor's recommendation.
- Make sure your doctor offers written instructions on how to use and maintain the nebuliser.
- Nebulisers may take 20 minutes to run a 2.5–4ml solution – the usual quantity.
- You should inhale all the contents and the nebuliser should be allowed to run dry – signalled by a spluttering sound.
- Modern nebulisers such as the **Sidestream** and **Ventstream** produce a fast and efficient drug delivery.
- Rinsing your mouth and face after using a nebuliser can help limit side-effects.
- Using a mouthpiece rather than a mask can reduce facial irritation and improve the amount of the dose that gets to the lungs.
- Nebulisers should be cleaned after use.
- Nebulisers should be serviced according to the manufacturer's instructions. An increase in the time taken to nebulise drugs indicates that the nebuliser is either worn or requires servicing.
- In children up to the age of about six, nebulised drugs can rarely cause paradoxical bronchoconstriction (page 109). So try MDIs with large volume spacers or face masks before switching to nebulisers.
- Some nebulisers work off car or rechargeable batteries. Others can be pumped by hand or foot – these are useful if you plan to travel.

Most doctors now carry nebulisers for emergencies. Applications outside of 'rescue' medication delivery include nebulised budesonide (currently the only steroid available for nebulisers), sometimes given if inhaled steroids fail to control symptoms – though this should not be seen as an alternative to a course of oral steroids. Less commonly, nebulisers are used for people unable to use inhaler devices adequately. Overall, people with asthma using nebulised steroids experience six times fewer the number of side-effects than those taking oral steroids.

There is a danger of becoming over-reliant on the nebuliser. Doctors usually advise parents to seek medical help if a child needs nebulised bronchodilators more than every three or four hours. But, according to a recent Scottish study, one in five parents used the nebuliser more than every two hours before seeking help – some even waited until the following day. Using a nebuliser this frequently suggests that the child is experiencing a severe attack and needs urgent medical help. It is advisable for anyone requiring nebulisers to see a respiratory specialist regularly.

Conventional nebulisers are noisy and bulky. However, a new nebuliser recently introduced into the UK – the **Omron U1** – is about the size of a mobile phone, weighs less than eight ounces and runs off batteries. Moreover, the Omron U1 is up to six times quicker than conventional nebulisers, although it cannot be used to deliver steroids. Many people with asthma will be attracted by its portability. You should be able to order the Omron U1, which costs about £300, from most pharmacists.

Adrenaline

Adrenaline is used to treat severe allergic reactions. It is rarely used in people with asthma. However, patients with brittle asthma (whose condition deteriorates rapidly without warning) and those likely to suffer anaphylactic shock (page 53) can benefit from it. These groups often carry an adrenaline 'pen'. This contains a spring-activated concealed needle able to deliver a dose of adrenaline rapidly and accurately. The effects wear off after 5–10 minutes, and the injection may need to be repeated.

An injection of adrenaline can save your life. For example, a study examined 13 patients admitted to hospital with anaphylactic shock, six of whom died. None of the fatal cases had been given adrenaline before they began to experience severe breathing difficulties.

The seven survivors had received adrenaline before, or within five minutes of, developing severe symptoms.

Adrenaline inhalers (e.g. **Medihaler Epi**), which look similar to an MDI, are less effective than the injection. However, adrenaline inhalers may be useful for some patients, health care workers and schools. If using an inhaler, you may be required to take 15–25 puffs of adrenaline within 3–5 minutes.

Adrenaline has a short shelf life – about nine months – so make sure you change your prescription before the expiry date.

TIP

If you or someone you know develops anaphylactic shock, seek medical attention **immediately**. If you live more than ten minutes from hospital make sure you have more than one pen. You could leave these in strategic places at home, in the office, or in the car.

Immunotherapy

Immunotherapy aims to desensitise a patient to a particular allergen. Introduced in 1911, immunotherapy is still widely used, especially in mainland Europe. An extract of the allergen is injected in progressively higher concentrations at a time when the patient is relatively symptom-free. Gradually, this strengthens the patient's response to the allergen, since a higher allergen load is needed to provoke a response. Doctors do not fully understand why immunotherapy works, however, and protection is rarely total. Another complication is that more than one trigger may affect an individual with asthma.

Because it exposes patients to high levels of allergen, immunotherapy carries a danger of inducing anaphylactic shock (page 53). As a result, in 1986 the Committee on Safety of Medicines, which regulates drugs in the UK, suggested that immunotherapy should no longer be widely practised. Since then, immunotherapy has virtually ceased in the UK except at specialist centres. Nevertheless, the Committee conceded that immunotherapy may be used where there is no viable alternative and patients' lives are at risk. So immunotherapy is used in people who develop severe reactions after being stung by bees, wasps and hornets. In fact, immunotherapy techniques using venom extracts offer patients 98 per cent protection from wasp stings and 80 per cent from bee stings. Other studies suggest that immunotherapy alleviates asthma due to cat dander, the house dust mite and pollen. However, immunotherapy is rarely, if ever, used to treat asthma without anaphylaxis.

Immunotherapy can be a daunting and protracted experience. In wasp venom immunotherapy, for example, patients are injected with increasing doses of venom over eight weeks – the 'induction phase' – and must then receive monthly 'maintenance' injections for another two or three years. Some doctors use more rapid induction schedules, but the risk of side-effects greatly increases due to the accelerated exposure to the allergen. Various physical conditions may make you ineligible for treatment: asthma and other illnesses, such as heart disease, must be well controlled, while certain drugs – beta-blockers, for example – will bar you from starting the course. Too much alcohol or heavy exercise on the day of the injection will increase the risk of an adverse reaction.

After the injection, patients remain under close observation for at least an hour. Emergency resuscitation equipment will be close at hand. Most adverse reactions, if they occur, emerge within the first 30 minutes. During this time, the doctor assesses any reaction at the injection site and measures peak flow, heart rate and blood pressure and takes other physical readings. Not surprisingly, this is stressful and many patients hyperventilate – breathe rapidly and feel dizzy – or develop panic attacks.

The risk of side-effects

So how great are the dangers? Research has been conducted all around the world into the likelihood of immunotherapy causing fatal side-effects.

- In the USA, the Food and Drug Administration, which regulates the safety and efficacy of treatments, received 35 reports of deaths associated with allergenic extracts used for immunotherapy between 1985 and 1993. Most of these patients suffered from asthma and, despite taking steroids, experienced attacks during immunotherapy. More than 90 per cent of the deaths occurred within 20 minutes, despite an adrenaline injection. This suggests that one person dies for every 1.4 million exposures.

- Doctors in Rome treated 2,206 patients with immunotherapy between 1981 and 1991. Of this total, 115 patients developed side-effects, which always emerged within 90 minutes. From these, 102 patients developed asthma with or without a skin rash. Four developed angio-oedema (a swelling of the skin and mucous membranes) and just one developed anaphylaxis.

- In the UK, side-effects emerged in 7.5 per cent of patients during the induction phase with bee and wasp venom, and in 2.1 per cent of patients given maintenance injections. In 81 per cent of patients side-effects emerged within 30 minutes, and in 92 per cent side-effects emerged within an hour. Only one in 200 cases required emergency adrenaline.

Despite rare occurrences of side-effects and sometimes death, immunotherapy can prove a life-saver among people who develop severe reactions to particular allergens.

CHAPTER 6

ASTHMA MANAGEMENT PLANS

Management guidelines

By the late 1980s, modern drugs treated asthma effectively. Despite this, the death rate continued to rise. To improve standards of care, specialists agreed a number of national and international guidelines for asthma management. These set the standard for asthma control and ensured that every doctor should be able to treat most of his or her patients effectively. Though there would always be some patients who fell outside the guidelines, they aimed to improve overall management.

The British Thoracic Society Guidelines were first published in 1990 and revised in 1993. Renamed as the British Guidelines on Asthma Management, they were updated and published most recently in February 1997 (the guidelines are summarised on pages 137–8). These British guidelines undoubtedly contributed to falling death rates, fewer admissions to hospital and an improved quality of life for most people with asthma in recent years.

The aims of management

Modern drugs mean that most people with asthma are able to live normal, healthy lives. Nevertheless, many sufferers have low expectations of treatment, putting up with daily wheezing and adapting to, rather than eliminating, their symptoms. Some may avoid exercise. The guidelines clearly set out the improvements that patients might reasonably expect to gain from treatment, sum-marised in the box below.

WHAT TO EXPECT FROM ASTHMA TREATMENT

- Abolish or minimise symptoms during the night and day.
- Minimise the need for bronchodilators.
- Restore normal, or best possible, lung function.
- Reduce the risk of a severe attack or exacerbation.
- Minimise absence from school or work.
- Maintain normal activity – including exercise.

If your experience of asthma treatment does not meet these goals, it is time to consult your GP.

To meet the aims listed above, the guidelines take a 'stepped care' approach to asthma management. The central concept is a 'ladder' with five different steps representing varying asthma severity. Your symptoms and peak flow define what step you are on and the number and dose of drugs. Most patients will probably be at step two of the guidelines. If the drugs prescribed fail to ade-quately control your symptoms, you move up to the next step on the ladder. Before moving you up a step, however, your doctor should assess your compliance – how well you are taking your drugs (see page 59) – and your inhaler technique. After you have spent 3–6 months at any step your doctor should review your symptoms and peak flow. If your symptoms are well controlled you may be able to move to a lower step. All drugs and devices mentioned in steps 1–5 are described in **Chapter 5**.

Step 1: Patients suffering very occasional symptoms may be able to use bronchodilators no more than once daily. However, some physicians believe that they should only take bron-chodilators a maximum of two or three times a week.

Step 2: Patients using bronchodilators more than once daily should take inhaled steroids: beclomethasone or budes-onide (100–400mcg twice daily) or fluticasone (50–200mcg twice daily). In children under five years the dose of steroids should be halved. Sodium cromoglycate and nedocromil sodium are alternative anti-inflammato-ries that may be especially appropriate for children under five years of age, though nedocromil sodium has not been formally approved for children under six years of age.

Step 3: Doses of beclomethasone and budenoside increase (800–2,000mcg daily), as does fluticasone (400–1,000 mcg daily). Doses of beclomethasone and budesonide above 800mcg or fluticasone above 400mcg should be administered using a large volume spacer. Alternatively, the dose of steroid can be kept the same as in step two and the long-acting bronchodilator salmeterol added (50mcg twice daily). If patients develop side-effects while using high-dose steroids, salmeterol or theophylline can be added and the dose of steroid reduced.

Step 4: If high-dose inhaled steroids still fail to control symptoms adequately, the dose of steroid remains the same as in step three and a number of other drugs are added:

a) inhaled long-acting beta2-agonists
b) sustained-release theophylline
c) inhaled ipratropium or oxitropium
d) long-acting oral beta-agonists
e) high-dose inhaled bronchodilator
f) cromoglycate or nedocromil.

Step 5: If these measures still fail to control symptoms adequately, single daily doses of oral steroids can be added to the high-dose inhaled steroids and long-acting beta-agonist.

Why are the new guidelines different?

Previous versions of the guidelines were similar to the latest draft. In addition to fine-tuning the protocol and including new drugs, the latest revision contains a fundamental change. In previous versions of the guidelines, the dose of steroid started low and was gradually increased until the patient's symptoms were adequately controlled. However, this meant that at each step about half the patients were using sufficient amounts of 'rescue' bronchodilator to suggest that they probably needed to increase their steroid dose.

As a result, the latest version of the guidelines advocates hitting the inflammation 'hard and fast'. This means rapidly controlling the underlying inflammation using high-dose inhaled steroids followed by a gradual reduction of the dose to the lowest level that maintains lung function and adequately controls symptoms. However, among children under five years of age there is no evidence that this 'start high' approach is any more effective than gradually increasing the dose.

In general, the guidelines suggest using steroids earlier in the natural history of the disease – e.g. among people with mild asthma. Previous versions of the guidelines suggested using sodium cromoglycate or nedocromil sodium at step two. Among the under-fives, low-dose inhaled steroids are now suggested as an alternative – although the latter remains the treatment of choice for children with very mild asthma.

Not everyone fits into the guidelines

The various incarnations of the British Guidelines on Asthma Management have transformed treatment for thousands of asthma sufferers. However, there are two important points to remember about these (and any other) guidelines.

Firstly, guidelines are designed to achieve the best possible care for *most* people with asthma. This means that there are always exceptions to the rule, and you may be one of them – so if you feel that your asthma is poorly controlled, consult your GP.

Secondly, the guidelines are dynamic. Just because you are on step two now does not mean you will stay there. Most doctors are prepared to move people up to the next step if their asthma deteriorates. But many forget the *quid pro quo* – moving patients back down if their asthma stabilises for 3–6 months. To avoid this, make sure you regularly monitor your peak flow, which provides an objective measure of lung function (page 72). If your symptoms are well controlled, discuss moving down a step with either the doctor or nurse running the asthma clinic. It is very easy to miss your review if you simply rely on picking up a repeat prescription.

You also need to evaluate your treatment critically. Despite the guidelines, a growing number of treatments and numerous educational initiatives, GPs vary widely in their management of asthma. While the guidelines have had a major impact, there is still some way to go before everyone is cared for in the most appropriate and effective way.

You and your doctor

What to ask your doctor

You should ensure you understand why your doctor prescribes any medicine. Asking ten key questions should allow you to understand why you have been prescribed a certain drug, how to use it and the risk of side-effects. Ideally, you could ask your doctor for written instructions or jot his or her answers down. Incidentally, most of these questions apply to any drug, not just asthma medicines.

TEN QUESTIONS TO ASK YOUR DOCTOR

1. What is the name of the drug? You should know both the brand name and the scientific or 'generic' name – e.g. Ventolin is a brand name for salbutamol.
2. Is the drug an anti-inflammatory (preventer) or bronchodilator (reliever)?
3. What are the side-effects?
4. How likely am I to experience side-effects?
5. How often or in what circumstances should I take it?
6. Do I need to take any precautions when I take it?
7. What is the correct inhaler technique?
8. Is there any risk of interactions with my other medicines, drugs that I buy over the counter from pharmacists, foods or complementary therapies?
9. How do I know if it is not working?
10. When should I return for review?

Self-management plans

Increasingly, doctors recognise that patients can play an important role in managing chronic diseases. This is reflected in the growing importance of self-management plans in asthma. Self-management plans formalise the relationship between doctor and patient, counter any misunderstanding the sufferer might have about their disease and help to alleviate poor symptom perception and feelings of helplessness – which undermine compliance (page 59) and contribute to anxiety.

The self-management plan is built around regular peak flow

readings (see **Chapter 4**) and a graded system of appropriate medi-cation use. Peak flow tends to fall before symptoms emerge, so peak flow offers an 'early warning' of an impending attack. So when your peak flow falls below a predetermined point, you increase your dose of inhaled steroid immediately rather than waiting to see the GP. A further deterioration may trigger a course of oral steroids or suggest an immediate visit to the GP. The final stage of the plan advises at what point you should consider going to hospital. The self-management plan works the other way, too – after your symptoms have stabilised, the plan may suggest when you can reduce your dose of steroid.

Some plans monitor more than peak flow readings – e.g. they enable you to chart wheezing and coughing, disturbed sleep, exer-cise tolerance and how often you use 'rescue' bronchodilators. All of these can provide useful indicators to your condition.

The graded divisions that represent peak flows are often known as the green, yellow and red zones, and vary from individual to individual. For example:

- Your 'green zone' may be a peak flow of 80–100 per cent of your personal best.

  No change in management required.

- Your 'yellow zone' may be a peak flow of 50–80 per cent of your personal best.

  You may need to double the dose of inhaled steroid.

- Your 'red zone' may be below 50 per cent of your personal best.

  You may need to start a week-long course of oral prednisolone.

Self-management plans can be extremely effective – you can mon-itor your lung function more frequently than any doctor. A study in New York found patients to be so successful at using peak-flow-based self-management plans that the improvement in their symp-toms translated into a threefold reduction in hospitalisation rates. Moreover, this improvement lasted for up to three years. In another study, patients increased their dose of inhaled steroid according to peak flow. This reduced the severity of the group's symptoms, and the number of nights they were affected by nocturnal asthma fell by 75 per cent. Nevertheless, the benefits of peak-flow-based self-management plans tend to be most marked among people with severe or moderate asthma – probably because this group has the biggest incentive to adhere to the plan.

The National Asthma Campaign★ and the Department of Health recently introduced an information card that helps asthma sufferers spot worsening symptoms and manage their condition. The cards are completed by GPs and nurses as part of the regular review of asthmatic patients. However, you should ensure that you also have your own personalised plan. You should be able to arrange this with your GP.

The following two chapters should help you manage your or your child's asthma more effectively, whatever the severity of the condition.

CHAPTER 7

THE THREE AGES OF ASTHMA

ALTHOUGH childhood asthma grabs most of the headlines, and most hospital admissions occur among children (see below), asthma can emerge at any time from the cradle to the grave. Indeed, recent surveys suggest that 6.5–17 per cent of the over-50s suffer from asthma. Yet even these figures may considerably underestimate the scale of the problem – many elderly patients are reluctant to come forward for treatment, so do not appear on the statistics charts.

Table 1: Hospital admissions for asthma in England April 1991–March 1992

Age (years)	Admissions
0–4	32,177
5–14	18,503
15–44	26,099
45–64	13,050
65–84	9,171
85 or older	619

This chapter looks at some of the problems encountered during the three ages of asthma. The population with asthma can be broken down into three age groups: childhood/adolescence, adults and elderly people. As each faces specific problems the chapter has been divided into sections accordingly; nevertheless, you will find useful information throughout.

Childhood and adolescent asthma

Q *How likely is my child to develop asthma?*

A The risk that your child will develop asthma depends on a complex interaction between his or her genetic predisposition to develop allergic disease – atopy – and the environment (page 50). This interaction is poorly understood; doctors do not fully comprehend why one patient might develop eczema, his brother hay fever and their sister asthma. Clearly, all these children have the underlying genetic tendency. However, they respond to the environment in different ways.

A number of risk factors increase the likelihood that your child may develop asthma or one of the other allergic diseases. The more of these risk factors that apply to your child, the greater the chance.

- **An immediate family history of allergic diseases** such as eczema, hay fever and asthma.
- **High levels of the allergy antibody IgE** IgE levels in newborn children can be measured by taking blood from the umbilical cord. Of the newborns who show high levels of IgE, about three-quarters develop allergies as children. By contrast, among those with normal IgE levels only six per cent go on to develop allergies. (IgE levels in umbilical cord blood are not routinely measured outside clinical studies.)
- **Boys are more likely to develop allergies than girls** Boys also seem to have smaller and more responsive airways as children.
- **A birth weight under 2.5kg** Low birth-weight babies are often premature. If a baby is born at under 35 weeks, its lungs are still developing. This leaves low birth-weight babies vulnerable to a range of infections and other diseases.
- **Early contact with allergens** A child born between October and January is more likely to become allergic to the house dust mite, whereas a child born between April and September is more likely to be allergic to pollen. Similarly, children born at times when fungal spores are common are more likely to be allergic to moulds. The difference in allergen patterns through the year may go some way towards explaining why siblings with the same genetic tendency develop different allergic diseases.

As a rough guide, during the first year of life children tend to develop sensitivity to pollen, cat dander, the house dust mite, cows' milk and egg whites. At about two years children become sensitised to birch pollen and between three and four years sensitisation to grass pollen occurs.

- **Exposure to smoke and tobacco** Passive smoking, as we saw in **Chapter 2**, is particularly hazardous to a baby's lungs. If exposed to passive smoking a baby is one and a half to three times more likely to wheeze. Do not smoke while pregnant or around your child (see page 193 for hints on giving up with the minimum amount of stress).
- **Viral respiratory infections** Some viral lung infections increase the risk of developing asthma and childhood wheeze (page 46).
- **Diet** The role of weaning and breast-feeding in preventing allergic disease is discussed later in this chapter.
- **Teenage pregnancy** The increased risk of asthma among the children of teenage mothers is probably not totally explained by social deprivation. Levels of the allergen antibody IgE increase during adolescence. IgE can cross from the mother to the unborn child through the placenta, and may make the foetus more susceptible to allergies.
- **First-born children** are more likely to develop allergies than their siblings. Children with older brothers and sisters are likely to have been exposed to viral infections at an early age, which protects them in later life.

Q *Can I do anything during pregnancy to prevent asthma?*

A There are no guarantees that anything you do during pregnancy will prevent your child from developing asthma. Nevertheless, recent studies appear to prove that events during pregnancy may partly influence the risk that the infant will develop an allergic disease.

Research is still underway, but some tests suggest that mothers exposed to high levels of some common allergens – such as the house dust mite, animal dander and pollen – or those who eat large quantities of nuts, eggs and milk may give birth to children sensitive to these substances. This is because the mother's diet during pregnancy appears to 'prime' the baby's immune system, setting up a pattern for allergic reaction in the child. As a result, pregnant women with a family history of allergies or who suffer from allergic diseases should avoid eating large amounts of nuts and other allergens, particularly during the last three months of pregnancy. You do not need to be obsessive: a small amount of nuts used as a flavouring in food, for example, will not do any harm. Moreover, if you restrict your diet too much there is a danger that your own health and that of your baby could suffer. You need to ensure you get enough calcium during pregnancy, for example. If there is not enough calcium in your blood to meet your baby's needs, the mineral is drained from your skeleton instead. This may leave you more vulnerable to osteoporosis – brittle bone disease – in later life. Dairy products, especially milk and cheese, are good sources of calcium. If you are worried about meeting your and your baby's nutritional needs, you may want to speak to your health visitor or midwife.

Q *Will breast-feeding prevent asthma?*

A There is no *guarantee* that breast-feeding will prevent asthma, or any other allergic disease. However, when breast-fed children are compared with bottle-fed babies, it seems that the former are less likely to develop allergies in general, and asthma in particular.

A recent study from Finland examined the incidence of allergic disease among 17-year-olds who had been breast-fed as infants.

- 54 per cent of teenagers breast-fed for less than one month suffered from atopic disease.
- 23 per cent of teenagers breast-fed for 1–6 months suffered from atopic disease.
- Eight per cent of teenagers breast-fed for more than six months suffered from atopic disease.

So breast is best. It is worth persisting at breast-feeding for at least 4–6 months, and for as long as a year if you can manage it. If you cannot breast-feed and allergies to milk are a problem, consider an extensively hydrolysed formula milk (see below). These may be less likely to provoke allergies than conventional formula milks, though they are more expensive.

Some babies may become sensitised to potent allergens excreted in breast milk. As a result, breast-feeding mothers from families with a history of allergies should avoid eating peanuts, tree nuts, sesame seeds and other potent allergens. There is no need to become fanatical about this, however. Eating the occasional trace of peanut, which may not show up on the food label, is unlikely to do any harm – unless you suffer from anaphylaxis (page 53).

Breast-feeding places a considerable drain on the mother. So you need to eat a healthy, balanced diet. Nutritionists increasingly recognise the importance of breast milk as the source of a group of fats known as the long-chain poly-unsaturated fatty acids (PUFAs). A high intake of long-chain PUFAs may prevent a number of ailments including heart disease, rheumatoid arthritis and asthma. However, both pregnancy and breast-feeding deplete your stores of PUFAs. To make sure you are getting enough, follow the advice below. If you are concerned, talk to your health visitor or dietician.

Q *Which formula milks are best and which should I avoid?*

A There are various types of milk on the market. You should be able to find the best one for your baby's needs.

- **Extensively hydrolysed formula milk** may reduce the risk of your child developing asthma. The protein in cows' milk needs to be relatively intact to provoke an allergic reaction. Extensive hydrolysation is a process that breaks down the milk protein, making it less likely to provoke an allergy. These formulas are more expensive than conventional brands. Ask your dietician or phone the manufacturer to find out about availability.
- **Formulas with PUFAs** The benefits of PUFAs are described above. In some parts of the world, baby milk manufacturers have to include PUFAs in the formula, although this is is not yet obligatory in the UK. You could check with the manufacturer.
- **Formulas with peanut oil** *Avoid any preparations containing peanut (also known as groundnut, or arachis) oil.* In 1993, French scientists reported that four babies with eczema seemed to be sensitive to peanuts. They suggested that peanut oil in formula milks might have triggered their sensitivity. Certain milk manufacturers have now removed peanut oil from their products. However, you may want to contact the company to make sure.
- **Soya formula milk** should not be used until the child is at least three months of age.

- **Soya, goats' and sheep's milk** should not be given to children under six months of age. These milks are just as likely as cows' milk to trigger an allergy.

Q *How can I ensure I get enough PUFAs?*

A You can ensure you are getting enough poly-unsaturated fatty acids by eating at least two portions of oily fish – e.g. salmon, mackerel and tuna – a week. This needs to be fresh or frozen: canning and processing deplete PUFAs. If you cannot stomach oily fish try taking a supplement; look for those rich in omega-3 and omega-6 fatty acids.

PUFAs may protect you or your child from asthma. Australian studies suggest that children who eat fish more than once a week are three times less at risk from developing asthma than children who do not eat fish regularly. Another study found that 31 per cent of children without asthma regularly ate oily fish compared to 16 per cent of asthma sufferers.

Q *What about hidden allergens?*

A There are some unlikely sources of peanut and other allergens. For example, some skin creams – including nappy rash creams – contain peanut oil (also known as groundnut or arachis oil) which is a possible allergen. Certain nipple creams may contain peanut oil, so your baby could ingest the nipple cream along with its milk. While any risk posed by these creams has yet to be proven and is probably small, you might want to avoid using them if you come from a high-risk family or suffer from allergic diseases yourself.

Q *How should I introduce my child to new foods?*

A When you introduce a young child to a new food, look out for certain signs: snuffling, wheezing, colic or a rash. If any of these symptoms occur, wait a couple of weeks and then try the food again. A second reaction suggests that the reaction is to the food itself, rather than the result of, for example, an infection – at this point you should contact a dietician. After a couple of days you can introduce the next food.

> **TIP**
>
> It is prudent not to introduce foods likely to cause allergies – eggs, milk, wheat and so on – until 6–12 months. Peanuts should be left until children are at least five years old to avoid the risk of choking.

Q *I think my child has an allergy to peanuts. What should I do?*

A Maybe one in 80 children are genuinely allergic to peanuts. Changes in diet may be partly to blame – until recently, children usually did not eat peanuts until they were quite old. Parents worried that peanuts could be destined for the child's nose or ears rather than their mouth and were concerned about the risk of choking. Peanut oil (also known as groundnut or arachis oil) is now increasingly used in processed foods and snacks, so children encounter peanuts at a much younger age. Indeed, about half of all peanut allergies emerge by the age of two, and almost all by seven years.

If your child really does have peanut allergy, this should be established by scientific testing under medical supervision. See **Chapter 4** for information on tests used. When a child suffers an extreme reaction to peanuts, which is rare, adrenaline can be used to treat anaphylactic shock (page 132).

Q *Should I restrict my child's diet?*

A If you believe the hype, certain foods could be responsible for anaphylaxis, eczema, nasal allergies, nausea, vomiting, diarrhoea, migraines, bedwetting, chronic fatigue syndrome, hyperactivity and several other childhood diseases. Widespread publicity of this kind leaves parents understandably concerned – in America, at least a quarter believe that their child is sensitive to certain foods. In reality, challenge tests (**Chapter 4**) suggest that only one in ten children reacts to foods, and that very few have true allergies.

Restricting a child's diet can herald several long-term health problems:

- underdeveloped size for the child's age
- low intelligence

- slow language development
- poorly developed reading skills
- social immaturity and behavioural disturbances.

A group of 5- to 11-year-old British children whose parents claimed they were intolerant to certain foods were found to be 1.5cm shorter than other children, even allowing for diseases that affect height, such as asthma. The greater the number of foods that the parents made their children avoid, the more the shortfall in height.

Food intolerance and allergies are real and distressing conditions. But remember that few children are allergic to foods and fewer still develop asthma as a result. Your suspicions should be confirmed either using a challenge test or exclusion diet – see **Chapter 4**. If you feel you must remove a certain food from your child's diet, you should talk to a dietician about making up the nutritional shortfall in other ways.

Q *Will vitamin supplements help?*

A Some studies suggest that people with asthma have low levels of vitamin C in their blood. Vitamin C is an anti-oxidant that mops up free radicals – by-products of metabolism that can trigger heart disease, inflammation and cancer. In chronic asthma, free radicals are one of the inflammatory mediators that can cause tissue damage (page 22). However, there is no direct link between vitamin C levels and lung function, and supplements of vitamin C and other anti-oxidant vitamins and minerals (vitamins A and E, zinc and selenium) have not, in scientific studies, improved symptoms. The probability of a link is currently being investigated. This is another good reason to ensure that you and your family eat sufficient amounts of fresh fruit and vegetables rich in natural anti-oxidants – at least five portions (each portion is about half a cup) a day.

Q *What symptoms of asthma should I watch for?*

A There are certain characteristics you should keep an eye out for (see below). Consult your GP if any of these symptoms seem to be persistent or are causing your child undue distress, and see below for more on coughs and wheezing.

POSSIBLE SYMPTOMS OF CHILDHOOD ASTHMA

- repeated attacks of troublesome coughs or wheezing
- a persistent, dry, irritating cough – which may be the only symptom
- wheezing or coughing that disturbs sleep
- wheezing or coughing between colds. Healthy children tend to cough for a few days when they suffer a cold
- shortness of breath after exercise or exertion.

Coughs and wheezes are endemic among young children. Though often a symptom of asthma, they should be treated with caution.

Coughing

This is the commonest asthma symptom in infants. Coughing, especially at night, following exercise or accompanying an infection may indicate that your child has asthma. However, 12–15 per cent of children at primary school cough persistently – especially during assemblies! Apart from asthma, pertussis infection (which causes whooping cough) and mucus dripping from the nose into the mouth are common causes of cough among schoolchildren. Nevertheless, one study found that almost three-quarters of children with recurrent or chronic cough were eventually diagnosed as having asthma. Doctors often fail to link asthma and coughing. They may label recurrent attacks of coughing and wheezing in children as 'bronchitis' and prescribe repeated courses of antibiotics. The danger is that this allows the inflammation to continue and makes symptoms harder to control. See also 'My child coughs continuously', below.

Wheezing

Wheezing is another hallmark of asthma. About a third of children experience at least one wheezing episode during their first two years of life, especially between 2–6 months of age – but this does not always signify asthma. Usually, wheezing episodes follow a respiratory viral infection and most cases are mild: after 3–5 days, the wheeze begins to lessen and the child returns to health after two weeks. Treatment often involves little more than tender loving care at home. Almost a third of these children never experience another wheezing episode, so doctors are correctly reluctant to diagnose asthma after a single episode of wheezing.

Q *My child coughs continuously. Does he or she have asthma?*

A A child with a chronic cough is worrying for parents – especially if there is a history of asthma in the family. However, coughing is a symptom of many respiratory diseases, and whether you should be concerned depends on the age of the child and whether they are recovering from a cold. Young babies, for example, sneeze frequently – especially during the first month of life. A baby's respiration rate is normally rapid and babies have a large tidal volume (the amount of air that moves in and out of the lungs relative to body size). Very young children do not have a well-developed cough mechanism, so persistent cough is abnormal and could indicate an infection or, more rarely, cystic fibrosis (page 66) or heart failure. If an infant has asthma, the wheezing is often difficult to hear but you should be able tell whether the chest is congested – a sign of asthma.

In older children, coughs that persist after a viral infection such as a cold has cleared up should be checked. Often, coughs are worse at night. Not only are the airways narrower then, but mucus drips from the nose into the mouth, triggering the cough. Some older children develop psychogenic cough (page 69).

Clearly, diagnosing the cause of a cough is difficult. However, asthma is one of the commonest causes of persistent cough and you should not ignore this symptom. Consult your GP if you are concerned about your child's cough. In some cases, measuring peak flow before and after using a bronchodilator (see **Chapters 4 and 5**) will help determine if your child has asthma. Nedocromil (page 101) is particularly effective against asthmatic cough.

Q *I'm sure my child has asthma. What should I do?*

A Consult your GP. Unfortunately, some doctors still underdiagnose asthma in children despite all the headlines and the best efforts of medical education initiatives. To be fair, a range of conditions can be confused with asthma, particularly in children, making diagnosis difficult (see **Chapter 4**). If you are worried, the following guidelines describe what to look out for.

- **Children with mild asthma** usually appear happy, do not necessarily wheeze when taking exercise or wake during the night, and eat normally. For these reasons it can be extremely tricky to detect the presence of asthma. Many children suffer from mild symptoms – often for many years – before asthma is finally diagnosed.
- **Children with severe asthma** frequently appear anxious, cough or wheeze during normal play, wake frequently during the night and have difficulty feeding. Persistent coughing and disturbed nights should be enough to suggest a strong likelihood of asthma to your GP.
- **Children with moderate asthma** show symptoms that fall somewhere between these two extremes.

If you are convinced that your child suffers from asthma and feel that your doctor is not addressing your concerns, try keeping a diary of the symptoms.

- note when, and how many times, your child coughs or wheezes
- note the circumstances: e.g. do the symptoms emerge only in bed? during exercise? when your child becomes excited?
- note any specific triggers your child reacts to (e.g. stroking the cat).

Your evidence will give your GP a much better insight into the severity of your child's symptoms and the possible causes of the asthma.

Q *Will my child grow out of asthma?*

A Some children eventually grow out of asthma, though even if symptoms clear up there will always be a tendency for the condition to recur. In many cases, asthma improves dramatically or may even disappear completely during adolescence, only to re-emerge in later life. So how likely is a wheezy or asthmatic infant to grow out of the disease?

Bearing in mind that wheezing is not always a sign of asthma, one study suggests that two-thirds of all children who wheeze before the age of three are better by the age of six. The respiratory symptoms termed 'wheezy bronchitis' tend to disappear in most children by 4–5 years of age and studies from Australia and the UK suggest that only about a quarter of wheezy infants still wheeze as older children or adults – although the severity of symptoms varies widely. (The risk is particularly marked, as might be expected, among smokers.) However, of those children who still wheeze *due to asthma* at three years about half either continue to experience asthma or suffer a recurrence.

Patients who grow out of their childhood wheeze regain near-normal lung function. How long it takes to achieve this seems to depend on how badly lung function is affected and the degree of bronchial hypersensitivity. So children who have poor lung function and very twitchy lungs tend to experience symptoms for longer.

For children with confirmed asthma, the outlook seems to be somewhat bleaker. Scientists followed 408 children diagnosed with asthma between the ages of 8–12 years for an average of 15 years. After that time, 86 per cent of women and 72 per cent of men still had symptoms. Other studies suggest that half of all children with asthma will still have the condition during their adult life. The over-all likelihood is that between a third and a half of childhood sufferers will grow out of asthma. In about 15–30 per cent of children with asthma, symptoms disappear during adolescence only to recur later. Nobody knows why the natural history of asthma varies in this way.

The statistics may appear weighted against your child. However, even if the asthma does not disappear this is not a heavy sentence. In many people, symptoms actually become milder as they age. And with modern treatment, most children with asthma live normal, healthy lives.

Q *My child keeps waking at night – what should I do?*

A Nocturnal asthma is a real problem, not just for the child but also for the parents who have to get up in the middle of the night to tend to him or her. The condition is often under-recognised and under-treated – many children wake wheezing or coughing several times a week. In addition, asthma can disturb sleep without the child necessarily waking.

- children with asthma are disturbed 19 times a night on average
- 50 per cent suffer disturbed sleep every night

As a result, schoolwork can suffer. Children with asthma generally show worse concentration than their peers – especially if their symptoms are poorly controlled. But those who develop nocturnal symptoms show worse performance and behaviour than those whose symptoms are confined to the daytime.

Fortunately, there are a number of options available to treat nocturnal asthma. Your GP should be your first port of call. He or she might increase the dose of inhaled steroid to help keep the underlying inflammation under control, reducing the risk of a nocturnal attack. Alternatively, children over five could take the long-acting bronchodilator salmeterol (page 112). One study found that when children with nocturnal asthma took salmeterol *and* increased their dose of inhaled steroid their sleep improved. The combination also boosted their concentration and creativity. Nocturnal asthma is a warning sign that asthma is poorly controlled, so make sure it is treated. See page 25 for more on nocturnal asthma.

Q *My young child can't use a spacer. What can I do?*

A Before the age of two, and sometimes up to the age of four, children are often unable to use a spacer correctly. Most over-fives can learn to use a dry powder inhaler (DPI) or breath-actuated inhaler, however, and children aged 10–12 years should be able to manage a metered dose inhaler (MDI).

You can encourage younger children to use a spacer in several ways:

- If your child is under two years, use a spacer and mask.
- Stroke your baby's cheek gently with the mask so that he or she becomes used to the sensation.
- Wrap your baby's arms to prevent him or her grabbing the spacer.
- When a mask/spacer combination is used, the valve must be open all the time, so hold the **Nebuhaler** vertically and the **Volumatic** at an angle until you hear a click and the mist containing the medicine emerges from the bottom of the chamber.
- Children inhale after crying. If your baby becomes tearful, do not be tempted to unhook the equipment but keep the mask over his or her face until the medicine has been delivered.
- You could administer the medication when your baby is asleep to avoid distress.
- Children over two can be taught to use the spacer without pressing the inhaler. Encourage your child to practise this.

- Decorate the spacer with stickers to make it look more user-friendly.
- Let the child hold and play with the spacer. Allowing the child to blow into the spacer is not going to damage it.
- The **AeroChamber** (page 125) can be less frightening for some children.

In younger children, one alternative is the **Babyhaler**. This is a small volume spacer – about half the size of adult spacers – that the baby empties in 5–10 breaths. A silicone mask fits over the child's face, which reduces leakage. The Babyhaler is easy to operate. In one study, almost 93 per cent of parents were able to use the Babyhaler correctly after a single instruction session. Moreover, most parents preferred the Babyhaler to previous devices they had used, which included nebulisers. The Babyhaler is currently not available on prescription. **Chapter 5** has more information on inhaler devices.

Q *My child's school doesn't seem to understand asthma. What can I do?*

A Schools are improving their care of pupils with asthma. In some ways, they have had no choice. As we have seen in **Chapter 1**, asthma is increasing dramatically among schoolchildren. Poorly controlled asthma can mean their education suffers due to days off school with severe symptoms and lack of concentration following disturbed nights. Clearly, it is important that teachers are well educated about asthma. Most children learn how to cope with the condition remarkably rapidly, even during an attack. So how can you better inform your child's teachers about his or her needs?

- Your child's drugs should be readily available in the classroom. He or she should have instant access to an inhaler at all times.
- Ensure that teachers knows what to do if asthma symptoms occur. They should know when and how to use the medication and any additional devices such as a spacer.
- If teachers appears dismissive, remind them that delaying treatment can be dangerous, may lead to a hospital admission and is terrifying for the child. Point out that even if another child uses the inhaler, they are extremely unlikely to come to any harm.
- Your child should remember to take the inhaler on school trips.

- In some cases teachers may have to remind your child to use the inhaler before PE, games or break. If your child does not like using their inhaler in front of other children see if a more private room can be provided. You may have to speak to PE teachers separately.
- Make sure PE teachers understand the difference between breathlessness and wheezing. Children with asthma who say they are too wheezy or breathless to continue games should not be forced to do so. This could be an opportunity to involve the help of the school nurse.
- Guinea pigs, hamsters, birds or rabbits may be kept as class pets. You may need to insist that they are removed from the class if your child is allergic to the dander (shed skin and fur) or urine of these animals.
- Teachers should be aware that fumes from certain chemistry and science experiments can provoke an asthma attack.
- Teachers need to know if your child has a confirmed food allergy. They should appreciate that food allergy is a potentially deadly medical condition and not a food fad. You may prefer to prepare a packed lunch.
- Grass pollen levels tend to peak between late May and the end of July, so children allergic to pollen may need to keep clear of flowering grasses during this time.

WHAT TO DO IF A CHILD HAS AN ACUTE ASTHMA ATTACK

If a child suffers an acute attack, you should:

- ensure the child takes the bronchodilator quickly and correctly
- stay calm and reassure the child
- encourage the child to breathe slowly and deeply
- help the child sit upright or lean slightly forwards – do not let him or her lie flat.

You should seek medical advice if:

- the bronchodilator has not worked after 5–10 minutes
- the child is clearly very distressed and unable to complete a sentence in a single breath
- the child becomes exhausted
- you are worried about the child's condition.

If a child has an acute asthma attack at school, it is important not to panic. The advice above on treating an acute attack is useful for teachers, parents and indeed anyone who is in charge of children with asthma. Make sure your child's teachers have been briefed on the above instructions, which could prove life-saving. You may want to write them down, or photocopy the box, so that there is no room for error.

Once an attack abates, your child should be able to be take part in normal school activities without any difficulties.

Q *My child gets very puffed after exercise. Is this asthma?*

A We live in an age of growing inactivity. Children often spend longer in front of the television, computer or video than in the park or riding bicycles around the streets (parents' concerns about safety also play a part in youngsters' enforced idleness). Deciding if you are breathless because you are unfit or because of your asthma can be difficult for both adults and children.

Breathlessness that seems excessive compared to the intensity of the exercise may indicate asthma. If this happens, consult your GP. Do the same if your child wheezes, coughs or complains of pain or tightness in the chest (some children with exercise-induced asthma also report a stomach ache). Remember that children with asthma may avoid sport to prevent symptoms developing – they should be encouraged to participate and taught asthma management instead (see **Chapters 6 and 8**).

It is important to identify exercise-induced asthma (page 31) for four reasons:

- exercise-induced symptoms may be the first sign that your child has asthma
- children with exercise-induced asthma may opt out of sport whenever possible, condemning themselves to a sedentary lifestyle with all the associated health risks
- recognising and treating exercise-induced asthma will allow your child to live a normal life
- wheezing after exercise may indicate that your child's control of his or her symptoms is beginning to deteriorate.

If you suspect that your child has exercise-induced asthma, pay a visit to your GP.

Q *Should I keep my child off games – or at least stop the football club?*

A Provided their asthma is well controlled, there is no reason why children should not take part in sport. Indeed, many successful athletes have asthma – see page 33. The all-round health benefits of regular exercise are undeniable. It improves lung function and staves off depression in the short-term and helps prevent heart disease and cancer in later life. Furthermore, children who do not take part in games may become moody and socially isolated. They lose confidence, which means they may be less able to fit in with their peers and cope with an asthma attack. There are therefore a variety of good reasons why you should encourage children with asthma to exercise while taking adequate doses of anti-inflammatory.

Certain sports are more likely to provoke symptoms than others:

- High-intensity sports performed in the cold may make asthma symptoms worse – e.g. 30 per cent of competitive figure skaters suffer from exercise-induced asthma.
- Swimming, gymnastics or downhill skiing may be less likely to trigger exercise-induced asthma than running, cross-country skiing, basketball or cycling.
- A recent Italian study found that aerobic dance improves lung function without triggering bronchoconstriction.

If your child is to play any sport, his or her asthma needs to be well controlled. Drugs can help reduce the risk of an attack while working out. When taken 15–20 minues before starting exercise, the short-acting beta2-agonists (page 107) prevent symptoms in 80–90 per cent of patients with exercise-induced asthma. The long-acting beta2-agonists (pages 111–2), sodium cromoglycate (page 102) and nedocromil sodium (page 101) are other alternatives. See page 173 for tips on exercising safely.

Q *My child wants to play a wind instrument. Won't this put too much strain on the lungs?*

A There is no reason why a child with asthma cannot play a wind instrument. It can be a good way to relieve stress. Indeed, taking up a wind instrument can even be beneficial for a child's asthma. Doctors recognised several years ago that professional musicians playing wind instruments have larger vital capacities (lung volume) than other musicians, so they asked eight teenagers with asthma who played wind instruments and ten teenagers with asthma who played other instruments to keep a diary recording their asthma symptoms and mental state.

There was no difference in the number of days both groups experienced symptoms. But the teenagers who played wind instruments were more likely to feel they could cope with their asthma than those playing other instruments – the former felt less irritable and less likely to panic or feel scared during an asthma attack.

Just as importantly, the teenagers who played wind instruments were more aware of bronchoconstriction and felt their inhaler technique was better. This can be explained in two ways. First, by playing a wind instrument patients' attention focuses on their lungs, meaning they are better able to detect changes in their lung function. Second, the co-ordination involved – musicians inhale deeply before blowing – closely mimics the skills required to operate a metered dose inhaler (MDI). There is no reason why a child with asthma should not play a wind instrument. In fact, they are more likely to benefit than come to harm.

Q *Are inhaled steroids safe in children?*

A Parents understandably worry about the risk of side-effects when their child takes any drug. **Chapter 5** discusses the side-effects of inhaled steroids in more detail. It is worth reiterating that, in general, inhaled steroids are safe in children. The fact that, even after years of research, many doctors are not convinced that inhaled steroids undermine growth highlights the subtlety of any effects. Overall, most studies suggest that side-effects begin to emerge only when the dose of inhaled steroids increases to above 800mcg daily.

The benefits of inhaled steroids are unquestioned:

- A group of children with severe asthma were treated for a year with 200mcg of budesonide using a spacer. They suffered less frequent and milder symptoms, used less 'rescue' medication and showed better peak flow (page 72) than a group of children with severe asthma taking an inactive placebo.
- The height and weight of the children treated with budesonide was normal and they did not suffer adrenal suppression (page 87). There was also no increase in the number of infections the children caught.

This is only one study of many showing that inhaled steroids are safe in children with asthma. **Remember that the dangers of uncontrolled asthma far outweigh the risk of side-effects**.

Q *What should I tell the childminder?*

A You might be worried if a carer with no special knowledge of asthma is looking after your child. To set your mind at rest, tell babysitters or childminders how best to take care of your child – putting your instructions in writing if necessary.

You could ask them to do the following:

- make sure your child is not exposed to known allergens
- make sure they know what to do in an emergency (see 'What to do if a child has an acute asthma attack', page 157)
- insist that no one smokes around the child
- tell the hosts of any party the child is invited to about any confirmed food allergies. You could offer to prepare some of the food
- adopt some means of letting you know where they are, such as a mobile phone or pager – you don't have to turn the latter off during meetings.

Q *My child feels isolated. What can I do?*

A The large increase in the number of asthma cases means that your child probably knows someone else with asthma. If not, the National Asthma Campaign★ runs the Junior Asthma Club for children aged 4–12 years. Some schools also support JAC groups. Meeting other children with the condition will help your son or daughter to interact socially and feel less isolated.

You should also encourage your child to participate in normal school activities and team games – there is no reason why children with asthma should be treated any differently from their peers (see 'Should I keep my child off games', above).

Q *I'm feeling stressed by my child's asthma. What can I do?*

A Childhood asthma does not only affect children – the whole family suffers. When a child is diagnosed with the condition, it would be unnatural if parents did not worry. They may focus their attention on the child to an extreme extent – even to the point of excluding his or her siblings.

It is, of course, difficult to stay calm during an asthma attack. But it is worth remembering three key facts to help you keep your fears in perspective:

- very few children die from asthma
- effective treatment allows most children with asthma to enjoy relatively normal lives
- some children's asthma improves as they grow older.

Do all you can to find out more about asthma to feel as in control as possible. Reading this book is a good start. You should also take time out for yourself, to bolster your stress defences. You could try some of the complementary therapies described in **Chapter 9**, which alleviate stress and promote relaxation. *The Which? Guide to Managing Stress* offers a number of other suggestions.

Q *I'm worried that my teenager suffers from asthma. What should I do?*

A Adolescence can be a stressful time for many young people, so having to cope with asthma is an added burden.

- Adolescents with asthma are more likely to abuse alcohol and smoke than those who do not have asthma.
- They are more likely to suffer a number of problems including loneliness, depression, feeling bad-tempered and unhappy about life.
- Teenagers may play down their symptoms – perhaps describing themselves as 'a little wheezy' when their FEV1 (page 76) is 50 per cent below normal.
- They may be reluctant to admit to chest pain during exercise in case it marks them out as being 'different'. Parents and PE teachers may attribute a poor sporting performance to their being 'out of shape' or 'not making an effort'.
- Some 20 per cent of teenagers now report some asthma symptoms, but about half have never been diagnosed as having asthma.

Part of the emotional problems are due to normal teenage angst. However, teenagers with asthma may latch on to their condition as the cause of their problems and enter denial (page 58). A desire to confirm that they are independent from their parents may also play a part in their rejection of authority. They may view themselves as almost invulnerable. As a result, how often they take treatment may suffer and they will be more likely to develop an asthma attack.

Surprisingly, adolescents who want to deny their symptoms sometimes get support from an unlikely source: doctors. Some doctors appear to be reluctant to diagnose asthma among teenagers, despite the fact that asthma is becoming increasingly common among this age group. For example, a Nottingham study suggests the number of 16-year-olds who wheeze has almost doubled over 12 years. If you feel the need to convince your GP that your teenager has asthma, as with younger children you could keep a diary of his or her symptoms (see 'I'm sure my child has asthma', above). This offers some evidence to present to your doctor.

Treating asthma during adolescence can therefore present special problems. The most important thing is to treat adolescents with asthma as individuals, and wherever possible to give them responsibility. Try to involve them in their asthma management plan (**Chapter 6**). Consider switching their inhaler to something less intrusive, if they are worried that it is hampering them socially (page 129). In other words, relinquish some parental responsibility.

Asthma in adults

Q *I've been asked to see the nurse. Shouldn't I see the doctor?*

A In recent years nurses have begun to shoulder more responsibility for asthma management, both in general practice and in hospitals. Indeed, management needed improving. In the early 1980s, hospital admissions remained stubbornly high. The UK experienced an epidemic of asthma deaths and patients faced unwarranted restrictions on their lifestyle. The increasing role of the asthma nurse combined with the British Asthma Management Guidelines (page 137) are two reasons why deaths from asthma are declining.

An asthma nurse's role is not primarily to change your treatment – although he or she may suggest alterations to the GP. Their main purpose is to help people with asthma manage their condition. Some specially trained asthma nurses hold an asthma diploma and most are trained to a professional level in asthma management.

They can help explain:

- asthma and methods of treatment

- how the drugs work
- why you should follow treatment guidelines
- why you should monitor your condition
- when to phone the GP or visit casualty.

Patients are more likely to accept this advice in the relaxed atmosphere of a nurse's consulting room than when facing a doctor. Indeed, the nurse is often able to devote more time to addressing patients' problems. Overall, asthma nurses provide a continuity of care that cannot be offered by GPs, junior doctors or consultants.

Q *Will being stung trigger an asthma attack?*

A Killer bees provide fertile grounds for film makers and headline writers. And in some rare cases, their reputation is justified. Each year 2–9 people die following a severe allergic reaction to a bee sting. Moreover, some unexplained deaths among the over-40s may be due to bee, wasp and hornet stings.

Sensitivity to bee, wasp and hornet venom is even more common than nut allergies:

- perhaps as many as one in five people develop severe local reactions after being stung
- skin prick tests (page 78) and tests that measure levels of IgE (the allergy antibody) in the bloodstream suggest that 15–25 per cent of the population are sensitive to bee stings.

However, not everyone who is sensitive to venom develops wheezing and the other symptoms of anaphylaxis (page 53). Only 0.15–3.3 per cent of people develop widespread reactions throughout the body that include symptoms similar to asthma. People with asthma who tend to have hypersensitive airways are particularly likely to be affected. Stings to the head and neck are most likely to cause airway symptoms.

It is important to keep the risks in perspective. Deaths from bee, wasp and hornet stings are rare. Wasp stings are twice as likely to kill as bee stings, but the latter kill at most one person in every two million. Over 70 per cent of these deaths occur in people aged over 40. If you are very sensitive to bee and wasp stings, there are measures you can take to avoid suffering extreme symptoms. Patients with severe reactions to wasp and bee venom may benefit from immunotherapy (page 133). You should also try to avoid being stung – wear shoes at all times, keep your arms and legs covered, use insect repellent and cover bins. If you are confirmed as being sensitive to bee or wasp venom, you may also need to carry an adrenaline injection with you – see page 132.

Q *Is there a link between the menstrual cycle and asthma?*

A Some women find that their asthma worsens around the time of their period, and a recent study has revealed that about half of severe asthma attacks in women occur before and during menstruation. About 50–90 per cent of women experience mild irritability and stress in the week before their period and one in ten women suffer symptoms severe enough to disrupt quality of life. Emotional stress can exacerbate asthma; pre-menstrual tension could have a similar effect.

There is some evidence that changes in levels of the sex hormone oestrogen may exacerbate symptoms. Oestrogen levels fall before the onset of a period; recent research also suggests that being treated with hormone replacement therapy (HRT) may slightly increase your likelihood of developing asthma (see below). Yet if oestrogen was a factor then Pill users should also be at increased risk due to oestrogen in the Pill – but this does not seem to be the case. At the moment, the significance of the role of hormones remains undetermined.

Q *Does hormone replacement therapy (HRT) increase the risk of developing asthma?*

A A recent study carried out in the United States that followed 36,000 post-menopausal women for ten years suggests that HRT may slightly increase risk a woman's risk of developing asthma. HRT delivers oestrogen and, usually, progestogen to relieve the symptoms of the menopause. The authors propose that the oestrogen absorbed may exacerbate asthma symptoms.

- women who used HRT for more than 10 years were twice as likely to develop asthma as the general population
- current users and those who had used HRT at any time during their lives were 50 per cent more likely to develop asthma.

These results need to be confirmed in other studies, however.

HRT reduces the risk of osteoporosis (brittle bone disease), heart attacks and strokes. Many doctors believe HRT's benefits outweigh the risks. Nevertheless, it is worth noting that a woman would probably need to take HRT for at least 5–7 years to markedly reduce her risk of developing osteoporosis. Shorter courses will lower the risk of osteoporosis and counter menopausal symptoms such as hot flushes.

Q *I have put on a lot of weight following several courses of oral steroids and can't get rid of it. What can I do?*

A Many people who take oral steroids find that their weight increases – partly because steroids increase the appetite. Inhaled steroids are usually enough to control the symptoms, and it is rare to require more than one or two courses of steroids in a single year. You should examine whether you are taking adequate doses of your normal inhaled steroid and beta2-agonist – check with your doctor. Anyone embarking on a short course of steroids should meanwhile ensure they have a supply of healthy food such as fruit and vegetables handy for when they feel peckish.

Q *Will my asthma harm my unborn baby?*

A Asthma is the commonest chronic condition among women of child-bearing age – up to seven per cent of mothers-to-be could have asthma. Women with asthma who want to start a family naturally worry whether their disease will harm their unborn baby. However, there is little evidence that either asthma itself or asthma treatments do any harm, as long as the condition is carefully controlled. Furthermore, severe attacks are rare among pregnant women.

- 30 per cent of women find that their asthma improves during pregnancy. Just as many women find that their symptoms worsen, or do not change.
- During a study of 500 pregnancies among women with asthma, 47 women suffered asthma attacks – no mother or baby was harmed.
- It seems that mild, rapidly treated attacks do not affect the length of pregnancy or labour.

Uncontrolled asthma attacks, typical of severe asthma, may lead to babies having slightly low birth weights. These attacks can reduce the amount of oxygen received by the baby, leading to excessive levels of carbon dioxide in the blood of both mother and child. This may cause premature birth and retarded growth. Other studies suggest that uncontrolled asthma may slightly increase the risk of pre-eclampsia (high blood pressure). Overall, however, the risk to your baby is very small.

TIP

- Avoid allergens whenever possible during pregnancy.
- You might want to discuss with your doctor or midwife whether you should avoid those breathing techniques during labour that involve taking rapid shallow breaths, also whether you should use your inhaler before breathing exercises.
- If you suffer an asthma attack during pregnancy you should go to hospital earlier than usual, so review your self-management plan (page 140) with your doctor or nurse as soon as you find that you are pregnant.

Q *I'm pregnant and breathless. Does this mean my asthma is getting worse?*

A Not necessarily. You bear more weight when you are pregnant. The effort of carrying the excess around with you can leave you breathless. In the early months of pregnancy many mothers – even these that do not have asthma – become more aware of their breathing, and many women also become breathless towards the end of their pregnancy. This is normal. Regularly monitoring peak flow and checking the variation between morning and evening peak flow (page 72) will give you some warning of worsening asthma.

Q *Are my drugs safe in pregnancy?*

A At least a quarter of mothers-to-be worry that inhaled steroids will do more harm to their baby than the asthma. The likelihood that asthma will harm an unborn baby is small. However, the risks from inhaled drugs are smaller still. Indeed, beta2-agonists such as salbutamol and terbutaline (page 107) can be used in high doses, both orally and intravenously, to relax the uterus and prevent premature delivery. The much lower levels you will absorb from inhaled beta2-agonists are undoubtedly safe. There is no evidence to suggest that inhaled beta2-agonists delay birth.

If you are using an oral beta2-agonist, you could consider switching. A large number of inhalers are now available and most people can find a device that suits them. It is best to discuss the possibility of changing therapies with your doctor *before* you become pregnant to avoid unnecessary stress.

Inhaled steroids

Inhaled steroids are safe during pregnancy. Indeed, women who stop taking steroids during pregnancy are some four times more likely to suffer an attack than those who continue treatment. This could be dangerous, as severe asthma attacks may retard the baby's growth and cause premature birth. Inhaled steroids enter the bloodstream either after being swallowed or through the lung, so it is sensible to limit the amount as much as possible by using a spacer (page 124). It is worth remembering that very little of the steroid that gets into the blood actually crosses the placenta and enters the baby's bloodstream – most of it is metabolised (broken down).

Oral steroids

Oral steroids are generally considered safe up to a least 45mg daily. As with inhaled steroids, enzymes in the placenta break down much of the drug – e.g. 90 per cent of prednisolone in the mothers' blood is metabolised. Nevertheless, some studies show that the risk of premature birth and delivering an underweight baby slightly increases in asthmatic mothers taking oral steroids and they have been linked to birth defects in animals. However, if a woman is taking oral steroids – especially when pregnant – she clearly has severe asthma. And, as noted above, this condition can cause premature birth and retarded growth regardless of the effect of any drugs (see 'Will asthma harm my unborn baby?', above).

Oral beta2-agonists

Oral beta2-agonists may trigger diabetes, a condition that pregnant women are more likely to develop. You might consider changing to inhaled medication – ask your doctor about this.

Theophylline
Theophylline has been widely used in the USA and there is no evidence of any long-term harm to the foetus. However, theophylline has been linked to birth defects in animals and it may cause the foetus to be hyperactive.

Anticholinergics
Anticholinergics can cause the baby's heart to beat abnormally fast.

Antibiotics
Many antibiotics, such as amoxycillin, are safe in pregnancy. You should avoid tetracycline, however, which has been linked to an increased risk of abnormalities in animal studies and can cause discoloration of the infant's teeth.

Q *Will smoking during pregnancy harm my baby?*

A Smoking early in your baby's life increases the risk of wheezing and also seems to impair the baby's lung function. A study of 461 Australian babies found that a number of factors increased the risk of the child showing reduced lung function. They included smoking more than 10 cigarettes a day while pregnant, maternal high blood pressure and a history of asthma. The message is simple: don't smoke during pregnancy.

Q *Will my asthma influence labour?*

A Asthma is not usually a problem during labour. If you take regular oral steroids, you may need to take hydrocortisone when labour starts and for 24 hours afterwards to cover the risk of adrenal suppression (page 87). The hospital also needs to be aware that you have asthma, just in case you need a caesarean section.

- having asthma will not prevent you from being able to have an epidural or use gas and air
- an asthma attack during labour is treated in the same way as any attack
- when discussing your birth plan with your doctor or midwife, include your asthma treatment.

Worrying about your asthma should be the least of your concerns when giving birth. There are psychological benefits to formulating a pregnancy plan – it will help you feel more in control and can go a long way to reducing your fears.

Q *I have asthma and want to breast-feed. Are my drugs safe?*

A Generally, there is no reason why women taking drugs for asthma cannot breast-feed. In fact, breast-feeding is very beneficial as it provides the baby with a vital source of nutrients unobtainable from formula milks. Very little of a low dose of any inhaled drug absorbed into the body enters breast milk – even oral steroids deposit only small amounts in milk. However, theophylline may cross into breast milk, leading to hyperactivity in the baby. If you take theophylline and are concerned, speak to your doctor. See also 'Will breast-feeding prevent asthma?', above.

Q *I think I'm developing occupational asthma. What can I do?*

A The first step is to ensure that you do really suffer from occupational asthma. There are three characteristics to watch for (see box below). Do not rely on memory – keep a diary and note where and when your symptoms occur and how severe they are. Remember you may use some of the same chemicals that could trigger your asthma at home and work – e.g. paints and cleaning materials. Moreover, the late phase (page 22) may mean that symptoms emerge during the evening, several hours after you were exposed to the trigger. However, if your symptoms worsen on Monday night and do not improve until Saturday, or if Sunday and Monday are your most symptom-free days, this could point to occupational asthma.

For legal and medical reasons you may find that your company asks you to undergo a number of tests to try and identify the cause of your asthma – including challenge tests (**Chapter 4**). If you feel that your breathing has become impaired because of an irritant or an allergen, you may want to talk to your health and safety officer and union. Resolving your problem may necessitate a change of environment within your company, or even looking for a new job in extreme cases.

HALLMARKS OF OCCUPATIONAL ASTHMA

- Symptoms begin after starting a new job.
- Symptoms begin after a change in work conditions.
- Symptoms are better on days away from work and on holidays.

Compensation is available for people severely affected by occupational asthma. Contact the Health and Safety Executive★ for a list of occupational sensitisers, or get in touch with the National Asthma Campaign★ who have produced a booklet on occupational asthma. **Chapter 2** has more on occupational triggers.

Q *Will asthma affect my chances of getting a job?*

A Sadly, some companies seem to be prejudiced against employing people with severe (rather than mild to moderate) asthma. A survey of 500 firms across Great Britain found that:

- 59 per cent of employers did not know what occupational asthma was
- only 19 per cent introduced health and safety measures to prevent occupational asthma.

Among people with severe asthma:

- 65 per cent report difficulties finding a work environment that does not make their asthma worse
- 59 per cent say asthma limits their employment choices
- 46 per cent regularly take time off work because of their asthma
- 39 per cent find their asthma makes holding down a job difficult
- 35 per cent are unemployed – 90 per cent of these blame their asthma
- 31 per cent report difficulties finding a job because of their asthma
- 14 per cent have been dismissed from a job because of their asthma.

These figures are disturbing. However, these people have *severe* asthma. It is true that uncontrolled asthma can have a devastating effect on daily life. This is frequently the result of patients not taking their drugs according to instructions. By taking advantage of the benefits of modern therapy and employing self-management measures (**Chapters 6 and 8**), few people should find that their asthma prevents them from doing what they want to.

Provided you take your medication regularly, you should not face prejudice in the workplace. Certain professions are, however, off limits to people with asthma due to the high levels of allergens and unacceptably risky situations such jobs would expose them to. For example, if you have asthma you should not consider becoming a welder, working with epoxy-resins, flour or wood, becoming a diver or joining the armed forces.

Q *Can I exercise?*

A Exercise is good for your lungs and the rest of the body. However, 40–90 per cent of people with asthma report some exercise-related symptoms (see **Chapter 2**). Fortunately, exercise tends not to cause the prolonged and intense bronchoconstriction that leads to hospitalisation, and unlike allergen-induced asthma exercise does not permanently damage the lung.

Make sure you warm up before exercising. For reasons that doctors do not fully understand, our lungs seem to become 'used' to exercise, and after continued activity the airway narrowing lessens. This protection lasts for about 40 minutes though the lungs will still respond to other triggers, such as an allergen. Warming up can be incorporated into a structured exercise programme, but it is obviously harder to warm up for running to catch a train! Even bronchodilators (**Chapter 5**) take 10–15 minutes to reach their maximum effect.

Some drugs can alleviate exercise-induced asthma:

- Take a couple of puffs of a beta2-agonist 15–20 minutes before exercise. This is the only situation in which you use a short-acting beta2-agonist to *prevent* symptoms developing, rather than to alleviate an acute attack.
- Sodium cromoglycate may prevent exercise-induced asthma if used 30 minutes before you exercise, though it is ineffective once you develop symptoms.

You may be able to use these without regular steroids if you only experience exercise-related symptoms, though most people with asthma still need regular treatment.

It is important to remember that a drug that prevented asthma while you played cricket during a warm July afternoon may not work for a cross-country run on a cold, crisp January morning. If symptoms persist you could try combining sodium cromoglycate or nedocromil sodium with a long-acting beta2-agonist. This combination should prevent almost all cases of exercise-induced asthma – you could discuss this with your doctor. Indeed, if you still develop symptoms the cause of your asthma may be another trigger altogether.

If you are a competition-level athlete and are concerned that your medication may show up on drugs tests, leading you to be banned, check with the Ethics and Anti-doping Directorate.* Most inhaled asthma medications are allowed by sports governing bodies. See also 'Exercise-induced asthma in elite athletes', page 33.

HOW TO EXERCISE SAFELY

- carry your inhaler with you while you work out or leave it at the touch-line
- if you begin to wheeze and cough, stop and use your bronchodilator
- avoid exercise on cold, dry days if possible
- exercise in short bursts
- exercise using just your arms or legs is less likely to trigger an attack than exercise using both.

Q *Will breathing exercises help?*

A Breathing exercises can be useful – many people with asthma find they benefit from meditation, yoga, Alexander technique and other alternative therapies. These treatments, discussed in more detail in **Chapter 9**, share a common theme of improving breathing technique. We have already seen that playing wind instruments improves asthma (see 'My child wants to play a wind instrument', above) – indeed, many breathing exercises use pursed lip exercises that involve very similar techniques. However, though many complementary medicines offer the twin benefits of stress relief and improving breathing, they are no replacement for inhaled anti-inflammatories. If you feel your asthma is well controlled enough to warrant a reduction in dose, speak to your doctor.

The controversial breathing technique known as Buteyko gained a great deal of media coverage during 1996. Buteyko is based on the idea that people with asthma over-breathe (hyperventilate). Most people breathe in 5–6 litres of air a minute: Buteyko practitioners claim that people with asthma breathe in up to 20 litres a minute, throwing levels of carbon dioxide and oxygen in the blood out of balance. Buteyko supposedly restores the balance. While some people benefit from Buteyko and other breathing techniques, there is currently no scientific evidence that they work. If you feel after a course of Buteyko that your asthma is well controlled enough for you to reduce your drug dosage, talk to your doctor first.

Q *Does salt worsen asthma?*

A Asthma seems to be a disease of the developed world: it is rare in the rural areas of the developing world, becomes more common in Third World cities and peaks among developed nations. This has led doctors to suspect that something in the Western lifestyle could be to blame for the rise in asthma.

Many aspects of a country's lifestyle change as its society becomes richer. One of these is salt consumption. The richer the country, the more salt people tend to use. In 1985, a study suggested that increased salt consumption may partly explain the increased likelihood of people in the West developing asthma. The study found that the regions of the UK that bought the most table salt were those with the greatest number of deaths from asthma – curiously, among men and children but not women.

Since then a number of studies have investigated whether salt intake increases the risk of developing asthma, with mixed results.

- Some studies suggest that increasing dietary salt intake enhances the airways' response to inhaled histamine (page 79).
- Another study showed that increasing salt intake reduces FEV1 and peak flow (see **Chapter 4**) and increases airway sensitivity.
- Other studies failed to confirm the link between poorer lung function and increased salt intake. Research by the scientists who first proposed the association failed to find a link between salt intake and asthma in men and women aged 18–70.

A more recent study confused the picture further. Researchers examined almost 2,000 men in the north of England aged 16–44 years: they failed to find a link between dietary salt intake and either asthma or airway responsiveness in shipyard workers or people living in rural Cumbria, but did find a link among men living in Newcastle. The study's authors comment that these contradictory results may simply be chance findings.

As no one has yet come up with a convincing explanation as to why salt intake influences asthma, the jury is still out – and likely to deliver a 'not guilty' verdict. Any link, if it exists, is weak; unlike the link between, for example, salt and high blood pressure.

Q *What can I do if I can't afford my prescriptions?*

A This can be a problem – especially for people caught in the poverty trap. Unlike some other conditions, such as diabetes, prescriptions for asthma drugs are not automatically free, although children and people on income support do not have to pay. There are no easy answers but you can take some steps to ease the burden. For example, you can buy a prepayment or 'season' ticket, which makes prescriptions cheaper in the long term – ask your chemist for details (you could regard the expenditure as a worthwhile investment in your health). You may also need to take a hard look at your budget.

Late-onset asthma

Q *How common is late-onset asthma?*

A In recent years, doctors have increasingly recognised that older people are more likely to develop asthma than was previously thought. Recent surveys suggest that 6.5–17 per cent of the over-50s have asthma. But even this may considerably underestimate the scale of the problem. Many elderly people experience symptoms for years before seeking medical advice or being diagnosed. An American study suggests that half of all over-50s with asthma experience symptoms for average of almost nine years before diagnosis.

In the UK, the National Asthma Campaign★ surveyed 768 people over 50 who had asthma. It suggested that 53 per cent suffered breathlessness and other asthma symptoms for at least six months before diagnosis: just over 33 per cent had symptoms for 1–3 years and 20 per cent had symptoms for over three years. Forty per cent blamed their doctor for not recognising the symptoms sooner.

The elderly are more prone to chest infections – indeed, doctors may misdiagnose asthma as chronic bronchitis, heart disease, COPD (page 175) or smoker's lung. However, many patients labelled as suffering from other diseases show marked improvements in lung function when they use a beta2-agonist (**Chapter 5**) – strongly suggesting that they have asthma.

Nevertheless, there are encouraging signs that doctors are beginning to treat late -onset asthma. A survey of over 750,000 people in the UK suggested that the proportion of asthma patients aged 65 or over being treated with steroids increased by 41 per cent from 1991–95. This was still somewhat less than the 54 per cent increase in other adults. Steroid prescribing is higher among the over-65s than other age groups.

The National Asthma Campaign has found that despite this advance, regular reviews of elderly people with asthma are not yet widespread. They reveal that only 32 per cent of elderly people with asthma have seen their GP during the last six months, while 45 per cent have not seen their GP in the last year; just 39 per cent are asked by their doctor or nurse to regularly attend for review. Most of those polled – 61 per cent – consulted their GP only when their symptoms became a problem.

Q *Isn't feeling breathless and wheezing part of growing old?*

A Many older people regard breathlessness and wheezing as a natural part of ageing. The National Asthma Campaign found that 40 per cent accept such symptoms as part of the price we pay for growing old. However, breathlessness and wheezing often herald asthma. So if you are experiencing these symptoms and feel you might have asthma it is important to consult your doctor – even if the symptoms emerged for the first time after your 50th birthday.

Q *Are the triggers in late-onset asthma the same?*

A Older people may respond to different asthma triggers than younger people. For example, levels of the antibody immunoglobulin E (IgE) decline in elderly people. As a result, asthma in elderly people is less likely to be triggered by the house dust mite, pet hair or pollen and more likely to follow an infection, exercise or exposure to chemical irritants – this is called 'non-allergic asthma'. Because of lowered IgE levels, elderly people are less likely to show skin reactions on skin prick testing (page 78).

The apparent increase in non-allergic asthma may result from long-standing inflammation in the lungs that leaves them sensitive to a range of non-specific triggers. Indeed, many older people with asthma may require relatively high doses of inhaled anti-inflammatories to stabilise their condition.

- pollution can be a problem if you suffer from other chest or heart diseases (see **Chapter 8** for anti-pollution measures)
- cold air can be a trigger – if cold air provokes your asthma, wear a scarf over your nose and mouth on cold days.

Q *Do other drugs exacerbate asthma?*

A Certain drugs may make your asthma worse:

Beta-blockers
These drugs treat high blood pressure, some anxiety symptoms and glaucoma. They act in the opposite way to beta2-agonists, which open the airways – so blocking beta-receptors (page 108) causes the airways to narrow. In healthy people, this narrowing does not cause any symptoms. However, in people with asthma it can prove fatal. Studies have also shown that beta-blockers can exacerbate the normal decline in lung function that accompanies ageing. Fortunately, alternative drugs can be prescribed for high blood pressure, anxiety-associated tremor and glaucoma.

Aspirin and NSAIDs
Aspirin and NSAIDs can trigger asthma attacks in people who are sensitive to a group of chemicals known as the salicylates. For more information, see page 37.

Speak to your GP if you are worried about any drug you intend taking. Do not stop taking your current medication without talking to your doctor first.

Q *What special problems are connected with treating late-onset asthma?*

A Most elderly people with asthma use and respond to their medication without any problems.

Older people are less able to notice their airways narrowing – one of the classic signs of an impending attack – than younger people. In one study, patients underwent methacholine challenge (page 79). All ages were exposed to what amounted to the same quantity of trigger, but younger people were considerably more aware of the symptoms that resulted than elderly subjects. Because of this, it is obviously important for older people to monitor their peak flow regularly (page 72) so they can stay on top of their symptoms.

Some doctors believe that beta2-agonists (**Chapter 5**) are less effective in elderly people with asthma. Certainly, some studies suggest that the number of beta-receptors in the body, which the drug must bind to in order to exert its effect (page 108), declines with age. As a result, doctors may advocate anticholinergic drugs (page 120) for elderly patients, especially those with COPD. If you feel your bronchodilator is not working well you could discuss switching drugs with your doctor.

Many elderly patients share the problems of poor inhaler technique frequently seen among younger people. About a fifth of people aged 75 or over suffer from some degree of diminished mental faculties. These people are less able to use an inhaler correctly and may need help from a relative, carer or nursing home staff. One study of elderly patients found that:

- 45 per cent actuated (pressed) the inhaler after they had finished breathing in
- 41 per cent held their breath for less than five seconds
- 30 per cent inhaled too rapidly
- 25 per cent actuated the inhaler before inhaling.

It is important to make sure that you use your inhaler correctly. If you currently have a metered dose inhaler (MDI), you may find a dry powder device or a breath-actuated inhaler easier to use. You should certainly use a spacer. **Chapter 5** has more on the inhaler devices available.

Q *How can I help an elderly asthmatic who is senile or demented?*

A The help that you can offer an elderly senile person with asthma depends on individual circumstances. Severely demented patients usually rely on carers in residential or nursing homes. Patients with some degree of senility who are living at home can, with the assistance of competent carers, use spacers actuated by someone else, nebulisers or – if all else fails – oral drugs. Side-effects tend to be more of a problem with oral drugs, however (see page 96), so they should be used only as a last resort.

Q *I have arthritis. Is there anything to make taking medication easier?*

A A third of elderly patients do not have the hand strength to operate a metered dose inhaler (MDI) – actuating an inhaler requires about 6lbs of pressure. You could try actuating a standard

MDI using two hands, or use a dry powder inhaler (DPI), which will not require any pressure. If external assistance is available, your carer could actuate your metered dose inhaler as you inhale the medication through a spacer.

Two aids are available to improve inhaler technique:

- **Haleraid** provides an add-on arm to your inhaler, allowing you to work a metered dose inhaler with the palm of your hand. It fits most, but not all, metered dose inhalers. The Haleraid also allows a metered dose inhaler to be fitted to a spacer (not snugly) – the drawback is that you still have to co-ordinate actuation and inhalation. Your doctor, nurse or pharmacist can advise you which inhalers the Haleraid fits.
- **Turboaid** makes the Turbohaler easier to use by the addition of a lever.

Your pharmacist can order the Haleraid and Turboaid. The Arthritis and Rheumatism Council for Research★ and Arthritis Care★ offer further advice and support for people living with this debilitating condition.

CHAPTER 8

HELPING YOURSELF

IT should be clear from the previous chapters that it is possible to manage asthma. You can consult your doctor if you suspect either that you have asthma or that your drugs are not working as effectively as they should. You can track your condition and predict the risk of an attack fairly accurately using a peak flow meter (**Chapter 4**). You can ensure that you or your child take medication in accordance with your doctor's instructions.

This chapter describes a number of steps you can take to help yourself. The key to effective asthma management is to educate yourself. The British Allergy Foundation,★ British Lung Foundation,★ Chest, Heart and Stroke Scotland★ and the National Asthma Campaign★ all offer advice and support. Perhaps most importantly you need to know when to seek medical help – either from your GP or from the local casualty unit.

The warning signs

It is important to be aware of the warning signs that herald deteriorating asthma – elderly people are especially prone to leaving seeking help until it is too late. Doctors estimate that better management could actually prevent some 80 per cent of asthma deaths, highlighting the importance of identifying and avoiding your trigger(s), using a peak flow meter to monitor your condition and seeking medical help when needed.

Three factors probably play a role:

- misuse of asthma drugs – especially inhaled steroids
- doctors still under-diagnose and under-treat asthma
- patients or relatives fail to appreciate the severity of the asthma and only seek medical help when it is too late.

> **WHY DO PEOPLE STILL DIE FROM ASTHMA?**
>
> Deaths from asthma appear to have reached a plateau in recent years. Yet despite the therapies outlined in **Chapter 5**, asthma still kills almost 1,500 people a year. Tragically, the vast majority of these deaths are preventable. So why do patients still die from asthma?

The epidemic of asthma-related deaths in New Zealand during the late 1970s and early 1980s (see page 110) allowed doctors to characterise patients at high risk of dying from asthma. The New Zealand epidemic was partly due to excessive use of high-dose fenoterol, which is now prescribed at lower doses. However, the findings – summarised in the table below – provide a salutary reminder of the danger signs that everyone should be aware of.

Asthma cannot be cured, only controlled. It is an unfortunate fact of life that some patients who record their peak flow religiously and take their medication correctly still suffer severe asthma attacks and end up in hospital. This is because peak flow monitoring and bronchodilator use are not infallible guides to symptoms and, moreover, anti-inflammatories fail to work successfully in everyone. If this was the case, asthma would be a condition of the past.

Table 1: Risk factors linked to an increased risk of death from asthma

Risk factor	Relative risk of death (ratio)
Hospital admission during the last year (as in-patient)	16.0
At least one emergency admission during the last year	8.5
At least three asthma drugs prescribed	3.0
Previous life-threatening attack*	3.8
Psychological and social problems*	3.5

* among people with severe asthma

When to arrange an appointment

In some cases, you will be able to wait a day or so before you see your doctor. Call your doctor to arrange an appointment as soon as possible if you or your child:

- wake wheezing and breathless during the night, or if your child wakes with a coughing fit
- feel wheezy and breathless first thing in the morning
- use your bronchodilator more than usual. At most, you should use a bronchodilator once or twice a day – any more than this suggests that your dose of anti-inflammatory needs increasing
- have a bad attack that is relieved only after several inhalations of bronchodilator
- develop a chest infection
- visit casualty because of a severe attack.

When to take immediate action

Call your GP immediately or go to casualty if you or your child:

- show a peak rate of less than 50 per cent of your best value
- have trouble completing a sentence within one breath
- are too breathless to eat
- are unable to stand
- become exhausted or confused.

If someone with asthma appears to be unconscious, call an ambulance straight away. Some doctors also suggest that you should call for help if your pulse rate is over 110 beats per minute (adults) or 140 beats per minute (children). Others suggest counting your breath – more than 25 breaths per minute (adults) or 50 breaths per minute (children) and you should call the doctor or visit casualty. However, heart and respiration rate may be difficult to measure when you are trying to cope with the stress of an asthma attack. Ideally, your self-management plan (**Chapter 6**) should dictate when to arrange an appointment with your GP and when to take emergency action. Regularly monitoring your peak flow and noting the number of times you use your bronchodilator will allow you and your doctor to agree on your personal trigger points.

So plan ahead. In some parts of the country, it may be quicker to go to casualty or call an ambulance. In other regions, especially rural areas, your doctor may be the quickest source of help. A talk with your doctor or nurse will help you formulate the most appropriate plan. Despite publicity about inappropriate call-outs at night, never be afraid of phoning your GP. Few doctors will object to being called out to treat an asthma attack.

Treating a severe asthma attack

So what should you do if you or a member of your family develops a severe asthma attack? While you wait for medical assistance you can take a number of steps to ease the discomfort:

- try to stay calm
- sit upright, resting your hands on your knees to support your back – do not lie down, which makes it harder to breathe
- try to take slow, deep breaths – leaning on a cushion placed on your lap may help, but do not squash your stomach into your chest
- loosen any tight clothing
- drink warm water – during a severe asthma attack you tend to breathe rapidly, which dries the mouth
- take high doses of beta2-agonist from a nebuliser or using a large volume spacer – you may need to take 5mg salbutamol or 10mg terbutaline.

By this stage you should be receiving medical help either at home or in casualty. The doctor may prescribe a course of steroid tablets or an injection to bring the inflammation under control.

Following a severe attack

You should regard a night-call to your GP or an emergency admission as a warning that your asthma is poorly controlled. If you end up in hospital or on oral steroids, it is probably time to review your treatment.

You should discuss several aspects of your management with your GP:

- **Are you using your inhaler correctly?** Poor inhaler technique reduces the amount of drug entering your lungs, undermining its effectiveness. Even if you learnt correctly at the start of treatment, your technique may now be imperfect. Many people 'forget' how to use their inhaler – especially if they have not experienced severe symptoms for a while.

- **Was your anti-inflammatory dose adequate?** Your steroid dose will almost certainly be increased temporarily following a severe attack, and you may be prescribed a short course of oral steroids. Recording peak flow allows doctors to assess how effectively your new treatment is working.
- **Was there an avoidable cause?** Some severe attacks occur because the patient runs out of medication or because their metered dose inhaler is empty. Others are triggered by exposure to a known allergen.
- **Did your attack herald the onset of brittle asthma?** This type of asthma – where a patient's condition worsens rapidly and inexplicably – requires a different type of treatment, so you may need to carry an adrenaline injection (page 132) to relieve anaphylaxis.
- **Did you respond correctly to the warning signs?** In many cases, what appears to be a sudden attack is heralded by symptoms that last for several days but are ignored by the patient or their parents. Do not feel guilty about this. Rather, regard it as a hard-learnt lesson.
- **Does your self-management plan need updating?**
- **Can you do more to avoid asthma triggers?**

Avoiding asthma triggers

Most cases of asthma are triggered by an allergen, a substance that produces an inflammatory response – e.g. the house dust mite, pollen and cat dander. The inflammatory response leaves the airways sensitive to a wide range of other substances, such as smoke, dust and even some perfumes. Clearly, to control your asthma you should minimise your exposure to asthma triggers.

In some cases, avoiding asthma triggers is easy. Ban smoking in the house, for instance, using the advice later in this chapter. In other situations, avoiding the asthma trigger can prove very difficult. It is hard to avoid pollen in the summer, for example. Nevertheless, there are some steps that you can take to reduce your exposure.

Allergen avoidance takes time, effort and, as you may have to buy special sprays or covers, money. But such measures can make a real difference. Since 1979, Swedish parents have been advised to follow rules similar to those given below. The results speak for themselves (see table).

Table 2: Sensitisation among Swedish and British children

Allergen/trigger	British children (per cent affected)	Swedish children (per cent affected)
Egg	49	25
Raised IgE levels	41	27
Milk	35	13
House dust mite	29	0
Cat dander	24	7
Grass pollen	6	4

Swedish children are more likely to be breast-fed, have fewer cats in the home, fewer bedroom carpets and gas stoves compared to the UK. All these factors reduce the likelihood of being sensitive to common allergens and of having high levels of IgE (the 'allergy antibody') in the blood. As the table shows, avoiding early exposure to allergens may reduce sensitisation rates in infancy. So how can you reduce exposure to common allergens?

House dust mite

You can take several steps to reduce levels of the house dust mite in your home:

- Dust regularly using a damp duster. This stops mite-laden dust from becoming airborne.
- Vacuum well using a high-efficiency cleaner. Remember that vacuum cleaning can make some allergens airborne, however, so open a window when you vacuum and ensure that the allergic person stays out of the room for a couple of hours afterwards.
- Service your vacuum cleaner on a regular basis and make sure any filters are cleaned and changed frequently.
- Keep the bedroom uncluttered to provide fewer hiding places for the mite and make vacuum cleaning easier.

- Cover your or your child's mattress and pillow with a plastic sheet. Older, impermeable covers blocked the allergen but trapped sweat making bedtime uncomfortable, damp and noisy. Newer, semi-permeable covers block the allergen while allowing sweat and moisture to escape.

- It is probably not worth replacing your mattress to get rid of the mite. Allergen levels return to those needed to trigger asthma within four months, and even new mattresses house colonies of the mite.

- Wash bedlinen at least once a week at above 60°C and pillows and blankets monthly.

- Keep the number of cuddly toys around the bed to a minimum – they are a refuge for mites.

- Place soft toys in the freezer for six hours once a week to kill the mite.

- Ensure that the house is well ventilated. A damp bedroom can increase levels of the house dust mite sixfold; window condensation and double glazing can triple levels. Airing the room daily halves mite levels.

- Mite levels are often highest in the living-room and in bedroom carpets and mattresses. Make sure these rooms in particular are well ventilated.

- You could remove the carpet from the asthma sufferer's bedroom and replace it with a vinyl floor covering and washable rugs. If you want carpets, consider synthetic carpets which produce less airborne material than wool.

- Mite levels are high in children's hair – according to a recent study of middle-class Brazilian children each scalp could harbour 2,000 mites. An anti-dandruff shampoo may help rid the scalp of dead skin cells, the mite's staple diet.

Acaricide sprays undoubtedly get rid of the house dust mite effectively: those containing pyrethroids, benzyl benzoate and benzyl alcohol directly kill the mite and those containing tannic acid dissolve it. Benzyl alcohol formulations kill 96 per cent of mobile mites and about 70 per cent of the eggs.

Various tests have been carried out into the effectiveness of acaricide sprays. In one study, bedroom and lounge carpets and upholstered furniture were treated every three months for a year. After a year, mite levels had halved and a year after the last treatment levels were still 26 per cent lower than at the start of the study. Whether this reduction enables people with asthma to enjoy improved lung function is debatable.

In another study, parents of children aged 8–11 whose asthma was triggered by the mite covered their beds with semi-permeable covers (see above) and treated the rooms with benzyl benzoate sprays. Scientists assessed levels of infestation and lung function in these patients and compared results with a similar group of children who did not take allergen avoidance measures. Combined use of bed covers and sprays was found to reduce mite infestation in mattresses to undetectable levels. The children whose parents used covers and sprays showed slightly improved lung function after six weeks, although there was no difference between the groups after six months. The authors of the study concluded that methods aiming to lower levels of the house dust mite were of only limited value.

In another test, parents applied tannic acid and acaricide solution to mattresses, pillows, duvets, blankets, household carpets and bedroom and living-room furniture and also covered their child's bedding with an impermeable cover. This had no effect on the number of house dust mites or on the symptoms of asthma.

It is worth noting that some of the studies carried out may have been conducted over too short a period to detect any improvements. The lengths of time involved mean that you may need to treat your home for 6–12 months to significantly reduce the allergen load in the atmosphere. As a result, it is probably prudent to ensure that you or your child are sensitive to the house dust mite before making any investment. The extent of the improvement you are likely to see remains an open question: medical opinion in the British Asthma Management Guidelines states that there are good reasons to suspect that mite avoidance measures may offer *some* benefit, but the scale of this benefit has yet to be determined.

Pollen

If you are allergic to pollen, try the following measures:

- Avoid long and freshly cut grass. Get someone else to mow the lawn.
- Keep windows closed on hot sunny days, especially in the

morning and late afternoon. Grasses release pollen in the morning, which rises on warm air. As the air cools in the late afternoon and early evening it descends back to earth.

- Grasses tend to release less pollen on cold, wet days.
- Keep car windows shut and, if possible, buy a car with a pollen filter.
- Wear sunglasses if you also suffer from hay fever.
- Beaches with an on-shore wind and mountains tend to have lower pollen levels than other parts of the country. However, pollen travels many miles in the wind so you are not immune from hay fever or pollen-induced asthma even in the city.
- Check the pollen count – this estimates the average number of pollen grains in a cubic metre of air – and avoid going outside on days with high pollen counts when possible. The National Asthma Campaign runs a 'pollen line'* in summer that is updated every two days.
- Many people find that their symptoms are worse on days when pollution is bad, which in cities tends to be worse on hot days with no breeze.
- You may need to double your anti-inflammatory dose during the pollen season.

Pollution

Pollution, as we have seen in **Chapter 2**, probably does not *cause* asthma. However, poor air quality exacerbates underlying inflammation in the lungs and can make symptoms worse.

Take steps to reduce your exposure:

- Do not jog in polluted areas.
- In the city, do not exercise with the window open.
- If you or someone in your family has asthma, try not to move to a home near a busy road, a power station or a site of heavy industry.
- Listen to air quality warnings. Try to avoid going into the city on days with poor air quality, or stay indoors.
- Wear a mask if you are exposed to pollution outdoors for any length of time, especially if you are exercising: your raised respiration rate increases the amount of pollution that gets into your lungs. Alternatively, wrap a scarf around your nose and mouth.

- You may want to double your anti-inflammatory dose on high-pollution days – discuss this with your doctor.
- Take action. If you feel you want to do something to reduce air pollution, consider writing to your MP or joining an environmental pressure group such as Greenpeace★ or Friends of the Earth.★ You can also help reduce pollution by taking public transport whenever possible and, if you have to drive, using unleaded petrol and buying a car with a catalytic converter.

Other triggers

You can also take steps to reduce your exposure to some other common triggers.

Animals frequently provoke symptoms in some people, so:

- if you or your child are allergic to animals, ban pets from the bedroom and wash your hands after playing with the pet
- if possible, wait until your children are older before getting pets
- wash the dog or cat each week; this dramatically reduces the amount of allergen that the animal releases in the home.

Cat dander can be especially difficult to remove – even if you remove the cat. The allergen seems to come from saliva, which is transferred to the fur when the cat washes itself. The small allergen remains airborne despite cleaning. Consider:

- getting rid of the cat and cleaning carpets and furniture to help reduce allergen levels
- washing the cat weekly
- using a vacuum cleaner with a high-efficiency filter around the room
- seeking advice from your vet.

Mould can cause symptoms in some people. If you or your child are allergic to mould, try reducing the relative humidity in the house (see below). Mould tends to die when the relative humidity is less than 50 per cent. Measures to take are:

- not drying clothes by hanging them on radiators
- opening the bathroom window after taking a shower or bath to let air circulate
- applying bleach-containing cleaners to, for example, visible mildew around windows (ventilate the area well).

Viral infections are a major asthma trigger. Common conditions such as colds and flu play havoc with the respiratory system, increasing mucus production and exacerbating asthmatic cough. You should discuss the following steps with your doctor:

- double your inhaler medication at the first sign of a cold
- consider getting vaccinated against the flu (page 194).

Should I splash out on 'anti-asthma' products?

Some doctors are cynical about the value of commercial allergen avoidance measures such as anti-asthma vacuum cleaners, air filters, ionisers and sprays. Devices and appliances such as vacuum cleaners do not have to conform to the same rules about safety, efficacy and quality as drugs. If a pharmaceutical company wants to market a medicine claiming to improve asthma, the drug is tested in a rigorous series of clinical trials. A manufacturer that wants to claim that their **anti-asthma vacuum cleaner** improves asthma does not have to subject the cleaner to such rigorous tests. To make matters worse, these vacuum cleaners may cost between £200 and £1,000 – more than double the price of a normal cleaner.

Some adverts claim that **air filters** are a sure way to prevent asthma, but this is not so. For one thing, asthma often has a multitude of causes. It is rare to be allergic only to cat dander, for example – although a filter may reduce levels of dander you could still react to food allergies, pollution and aspirin. Similarly, one study claimed that high-temperature **steam cleaning** can reduce levels of the mite in carpets by about 64 per cent. But this reduction is probably insufficient to offer any real clinical benefits. **Ionisers** have also been reported to have miraculous properties – yet there is no evidence that they have any effect on asthma. There is some controversy over whether **acaricide sprays** (see page 186) actually improve symptoms.

How to quit smoking

Tobacco is the greatest single preventative threat to health in general and asthma in particular. Smoking accounts for 87 per cent of deaths from lung cancer; 82 per cent of deaths from COPD (page 65); 21 per cent of deaths from coronary heart disease; and 18 per cent of deaths from strokes. Indeed, smoking is the leading cause of premature death in the UK. Yet despite the dangers many people with asthma smoke.

Quitting smoking can make a dramatic difference to your lifespan: a year after quitting, your risk of developing heart disease halves. Within 15 years your risk of dying from heart disease approaches that among non-smokers and your risk of death from lung cancer, COPD and strokes also declines, albeit more slowly. After 10–14 years have passed, your lung function and risk of dying from cancer will be only slightly worse than among lifelong non-smokers. This should be incentive enough to give up. However, people with asthma have an extra incentive to quit.

Over time, smokers who have asthma find that their symptoms become less reversible – their bronchodilator and anti-inflammatory gradually become less effective. Stopping smoking is, however, especially difficult for people with asthma. Many people with asthma find that their symptoms worsen in the days and weeks after they quit. It takes time for the lungs to change from being unhealthily drenched in tobacco-laden mucus to relatively healthy cells – as the lung changes, the cells become raw and sensitive. Consequently, some doctors advise smokers to double their dose of anti-inflammatory for the first month after giving up.

Passive smoking and children

If you don't want to give up for the sake of your own health, give up for the sake of your children's. As mentioned earlier, passive smoking exacerbates asthma symptoms (page 45) and several studies underline the effect on children's health. In one experiment doctors measured levels of coetine – a chemical produced when the body breaks down (metabolises) nicotine – in the urine of children with asthma.

- compared to those raised in non-smoking homes, children exposed to one person's smoke excreted more than double the amount of coetine
- in children exposed to more than one source of smoke, coetine levels were over ten times higher.

Smoking when pregnant can harm your baby (see page 169), and lung function in children declines as exposure increases – not to mention the additional risks of asthma attacks, carcinogens, heart disease, brain tumours and eczema. Giving up will make your children both healthier and happier. So if you don't quit smoking for yourself, quit for your family – otherwise, do your child's lungs a favour and smoke outside.

The problem with nicotine

Perhaps because it is legal, most people underestimate the risk of nicotine addiction. However, casual smokers are more likely to become long-term users than occasional users of cocaine or even morphine are to become addicts. They are also more likely to become addicted than social drinkers are to become alcohol abusers. Nicotine shares many of the actions on the brain that make cocaine addictive. Indeed, nicotine produces long-lasting changes in the brain that increase the likelihood of tolerance and dependence.

Compared to the rest of the population, people with anxiety disorders are twice as likely to smoke and alcoholics are almost five times more likely to smoke. Sixty per cent of smokers report suffering from depression sometime during their life.

Ironically, the most effective (and therefore the most lethal and addictive) nicotine delivery systems – cigarettes, cigars and pipe tobacco – are widely available from supermarkets, newsagents and vending machines. Other nicotine delivery systems – those designed to help wean people off the weed, such as nicotine patches – are available only from pharmacists or on a doctor's prescription.

How effective are nicotine replacement therapies?

Nicotine replacement therapies certainly aren't cheap – indeed, nicotine patches cost about as much per week as the average smoker spends on cigarettes. Both nicotine gum and patches can only help you to quit provided you are motivated to begin with.

A survey of 14 trials of nicotine gum suggested that 25 per cent of users abstained from smoking after using the gum compared to 22 per cent who chewed a placebo gum. Trials in smoking clinics suggested that 36 per cent of people using nicotine chewing gum abstained from lighting up, compared to 23 per cent who used a placebo. Patches appear to be relatively more effective. Up to 21 per cent of volunteers using patches were able to abstain from smoking compared to about 10 per cent of those who applied a placebo patch. The relatively high rate of placebo successes demonstrates the key role willpower plays. Nicotine patches can roughly double your chance of quitting, provided you want to succeed.

Some people using nicotine replacement therapies complain of side-effects. Nicotine gums can cause gastrointestinal disturbances including hiccups, mouth discomfort, heartburn and nausea. Patches bypass these side-effects although they may still cause headaches, dizziness, fatigue and skin reactions. If these develop, talk to your pharmacist – another treatment may cause less discomfort.

Be realistic

Nicotine is so addictive that it can undermine the strongest will, so it is important to be realistic. Only 40 per cent of smokers succeed in giving up totally. Often smokers take several attempts before finally succeeding. Nevertheless, you can enhance your chances of quitting.

- Be prepared to feel slightly depressed or irritable after you stop smoking. Three-quarters of smokers with a history of depression suffer a recurrence after they stop, and about 30 per cent of people with no previous experience of depression report a low mood during the first week after giving up.
- Ask your family for support and understanding. Most families are more than happy to put up with a few days of grouchiness if it helps you to quit. It will help even more if you spend some of the money you save on cigarettes on a treat for the family.
- Try to identify your smoking triggers. Do you smoke when you are tense? When you are bored? Only after meals? Try keeping a diary for a couple of weeks noting when, where and how you feel when you light up. Identifying your smoking triggers may help you to avoid them.
- So-called 'sedative smokers' smoke to calm down. 'Stimulant smokers' use cigarettes like cups of coffee to increase their arousal and enhance their performance. Relaxation techniques (see **Chapter 9**) and herbal stress remedies tend to be most effective in sedative smokers. Stimulant smokers could substitute coffee, diet cola or energy drinks.

- Don't make things difficult for yourself. Sit in no-smoking areas in restaurants and ask friends not to smoke in front of you.
- Chewing sugar-free gum may help you resist the urge to smoke.
- Aim to spend at least some of the money you save on yourself, such as a holiday.
- Quitline★ and Action on Smoking and Health (ASH)★ offer advice, information and support.

It's worth making the effort. In time your lungs will begin to heal, which will reduce the risk of an exacerbation. You will be better able to control your asthma, and you will reduce the risk to your children's health.

TIP

Before giving up, get other conditions treated first – especially psychological or stress-related disorders. Anxiety, depression and alcohol abuse all increase your risk of smoking in the first place, make quitting harder and a relapse more likely (failing to quit could increase your stress levels). If you are having problems, consult your GP to help manage your underlying condition.

Influenza

It's easy to underestimate influenza. To most people, a bout of the flu is an excuse for a couple of days off work and is synonymous with a heavy cold. However, influenza kills thousands of people every year. Vaccines could prevent three-quarters of these deaths but despite this less than half the 'at risk' population, which includes people with asthma (see below), are vaccinated. Influenza is dangerous to people with asthma because, like any lung infection, it causes the condition to worsen.

Influenza probably arose while animals were being domesticated between about 2000 and 5000 BC. Influenza mutates as it crosses between animals and humans and *vice versa*. The close contact between humans and farm animals made it relatively easy for influenza mutations to jump the species barrier and also explains why many of the new strains arise in the developing world, where humans and animals still live in close proximity. These mutations are responsible for the large number of flu strains worldwide, which occasionally develop into pandemics affecting millions of people across several countries. The earliest definite reports of influenza date from AD 1387, while the first pandemic took place in the sixteenth century. Pandemics have swept the world periodically ever since – seven during this century alone.

During a pandemic the death toll from influenza is immense. 'Spanish' or 'swine' flu killed 20 million people worldwide in 1918. During the 1989–90 epidemic, influenza caused 29,000 excess deaths in the UK alone. Three years later another flu epidemic accounted for 13,000 deaths. Influenza strikes hardest against the most vulnerable people in the community – the elderly, people with asthma and patients suffering from heart, endocrine or kidney diseases. Even in a non-epidemic year, the complications of influenza kill 3,000–4,000 people in the UK.

Vaccination reduces the toll exerted by influenza. It prevents up to 65 per cent of deaths from influenza-related respiratory illnesses and cuts hospital admissions among diabetics by 79 per cent, for example. In elderly people, it reduces the risk of hospitalisation for pneumonia and influenza by up to 57 per cent and lowers the general death rate by up to 54 per cent. The benefits are less marked in younger people, but all asthmatics – especially those taking high-dose inhaled or oral steroids – should make sure they are vaccinated every year.

Who should be vaccinated?

The government's current vaccination strategy reduces the population's risk of being infected with influenza by 70–80 per cent. The programme targets people at high risk of developing complications if they contract the virus: about 83 per cent of people who die from flu are over 75 years old, for example. Most of this group also have serious concurrent conditions. About 51 per cent of elderly people fall into at least one high-risk group. So the government suggests vaccinating elderly people in particular, and – from six months old – people who suffer from:

- asthma, bronchitis and chronic lung conditions that cause breathlessness

- immunosuppressed patients, e.g. those taking oral steroids or chemotherapy
- chronic heart disease
- kidney disease
- chronic endocrine disorders, e.g. diabetes mellitus
- elderly people in residential homes and other long-stay accommodation.

In other words all asthma sufferers, but especially older people and those taking oral (and probably high-dose inhaled) steroids should be vaccinated. The government does not currently recommend routine vaccination of fit children and adults. However, if asked many GPs will vaccinate the carers of people with high-risk diseases. This means that if a carer is exposed to the virus he or she is less likely to infect the patient. If you care for someone with severe asthma you may therefore want to consider a flu jab.

The vaccine takes 10–14 days to offer protection and immunity lasts for about six months. As influenza is rare before the middle of November, the ideal time for vaccination is October or early November. Immunity lasts throughout the winter and the vaccine's composition changes each year to reflect microbiologists' best guess at the strains likely to cause flu during the winter.

An opportunity not to be missed

Despite clear indications of the benefits of flu vaccination and the annual government circular reminding GPs to vaccinate at-risk groups, only 40–50 per cent of 'at risk' groups receive the necessary injection. Even among people living in residential and nursing homes, just 40 per cent of residents receive vaccine. There seems to be little reason for this shortfall.

Patients are unlikely to suffer side-effects, for example. In one trial, 336 elderly people received either active vaccine followed two weeks later by a placebo or *vice versa*. The study did not record any difference in the number of patients reporting side-effects from either group, or a reduced ability in participants to perform normal daily tasks. Side-effects are not common. Occasionally, recipients suffer soreness at the injection site. More rarely, fevers, malaise and muscle pains develop 6–12 hours after immunisation and can last for up to 48 hours. You should not worry that flu vaccination can trigger influenza: the vaccine contains inactivated viruses. So the message for asthma sufferers is clear: get vaccinated!

IMPORTANT

You should **not** be given the influenza vaccine if:

- you are allergic to chickens or eggs (the vaccine is grown on hen's eggs)
- you have a feverish illness such as a cold – the injection should be postponed until you have recovered.

CHAPTER 9

ASTHMA AND COMPLEMENTARY THERAPIES

PEOPLE with asthma are increasingly turning to complementary therapies in the hope that these will reduce the amount of medication they use, especially if they are taking high-dose or oral steroids. Complementary treatments can be effective and some therapies may directly improve asthma: indeed, the National Asthma Campaign⋆ recently appointed its first adviser on complementary therapies.

Although asthma is not caused by nerves, heightened emotions and stress can trigger an attack. Most complementary therapies reduce stress and anxiety and can help you to deal with the depression and anxiety that follow in the wake of a severe attack. Bolstering your stress defences also makes coping with an attack easier.

In this chapter we look some of the leading therapies that may directly benefit asthma. As many of the complementary therapies involve breath control, it is probably wise to ensure that your asthma is well controlled before you embark on the course. You may want to speak to your GP – although don't be put off if he or she regards your idea with a certain scepticism.

Most people who try complementary therapies find that their symptoms improve after a few weeks or months, partly perhaps because the neuroendocrine system – the two-way information superhighway between the body and the brain – reduces inflammation levels when you are under less stress. Nevertheless, you should keep your bronchodilator handy, continue to monitor your peak flow (**Chapter 4**) and take your anti-inflammatory treatment correctly. If your lung function improves, you will be in a position to consult your doctor about lessening your dose. Under current treatment guidelines, doctors should begin to reduce your anti-inflammatory dose to the lowest amount that will control your symptoms after your asthma has been stable for 3–6 months.

It is important to find the therapy that suits you and your lifestyle. *The Which? Guide to Complementary Medicine* and *The Which? Guide to Managing Stress* explore complementary therapies in more detail. The Council for Complementary and Alternative Medicine,★ the Institute for Complementary Medicine★ and the British Complementary Medicine Association★ are umbrella organisations for complementary and alternative therapies. They should provide you with further information and advice.

IMPORTANT

None of the following therapies will enable you to throw your inhalers away: they are *complementary* to conventional medicine rather than *alternatives*. You should keep using your asthma medication unless your doctor advises otherwise.

Acupuncture

Acupuncture, one of the oldest medical treatments, remains one of the most widely used worldwide. Archaeologists uncovered stone acupuncture needles dating from 10,000 BC and the first acupuncture texts were written over 2,000 years ago. Now over three million healers practise acupuncture worldwide, most of these in Asia. Although acupuncture's roots lie deep in Eastern philosophy, it is increasingly used by Western doctors and complementary practitioners. Nevertheless, there are some important differences between Western and Eastern approaches.

Chinese acupuncture

The Chinese believe that every organ, process and action of the human body contains *qi* or 'chi' (also translated as 'ki'), a vital energy. Chi flows along 12 meridians running through the body that link the internal organs. Acupuncturists believe diseases arise when stress, anxiety, fear, grief, infections or trauma disturb the flow of chi. Acupuncture aims to balance the flow of chi along these meridians and so prevent and treat illness.

Because chi flows along meridians, acupuncture needles inserted into one part of your body may influence organs some distance away. So to treat asthma, the acupuncturist may needle the end of the meridian for the lungs, for example. Alternatively, they may needle two points on the back – called the soothing asthma points – or a point at the top of the breast bone (the *xi* cleft or *din chaun* point). This, in about half the patients treated, substantially alleviates symptoms. Studies show that needling the *din chaun* point will reduce asthmatic wheezing, whereas needling non-specific points around the body offers no benefit. However, despite offering improvement, acupuncture cannot cure asthma.

Because acupuncturists believe that the meridians convey so much information, by feeling your pulse Chinese doctors can tell far more about your health than just your heart rate. However, pulse diagnosis is backed by questions about your lifestyle, medical history, diet, sleep patterns and emotions that allow the practitioner to develop a picture of you and your asthma.

Western acupuncture

Western medical acupuncturists take a different approach – they look for trigger points. When pressed, trigger points evoke a sensation in another part of the body, usually pain. Injury, strain, stress, damp, cold, infection and muscle tension can cause trigger points. For example, when we are stressed we tense our muscles. Over time, muscle tension leads to trigger points, which in turn may establish other trigger points. Medical acupuncturists insert a needle into these trigger points.

Trigger points can also be warmed using moxa, a herb that burns without producing an intense heat – known as moxibustion. Moxa (or common mugwort) is applied either directly to the skin or to the end of the acupuncture needle. In other cases, the needle is stimulated using an electrical current.

Practitioners may also press or tap the acupuncture point, a technique known as acupressure.

Another traditional therapy, known as cupping, is often used by acupuncture practitioners to treat asthma. This involves a small amount of cotton wool that has been soaked in alcohol being burnt inside a cup. This is placed over the appropriate area of the body, creating a vacuum that sucks the flesh into the cup. Traditional practitioners believe that cupping is especially appropriate for asthma, bronchitis and some other conditions.

Is acupuncture effective?

Conventional doctors regard acupuncture as safe and effective – but only for reversible conditions, such as pain. According to conventional medical theory, acupuncture works by stimulating the release of natural opioid pain-killers. Acupuncture has been used on detoxification programmes, to provide pain relief in childbirth and to treat people suffering from nausea due to chemotherapy. However, most doctors are more sceptical about whether acupuncture offers any real benefit in chronic diseases such as asthma.

In contrast, acupuncturists believe that acupuncture helps a wide range of conditions including anxiety, allergies, migraine, high blood pressure and menstrual problems by re-balancing the physical, spiritual and emotional aspects of a person's character. This stimulates the body's innate healing abilities. Arguments between conventional doctors and traditional acupuncturists now focus on what conditions acupuncture can treat successfully rather than whether or not it works, however.

The British Acupuncture Council,★ which governs acupuncture in the UK, can supply a list of qualified practitioners in your area. Many GPs now offer acupuncture – usually only for pain relief. Make sure that whoever treats you uses sterile needles.

Alexander technique

At around the end of the last century, the Australian actor Frederick Matthias Alexander began experiencing serious voice problems, which doctors could not alleviate. Alexander noticed that when he spoke he pulled his head back. He also inhaled when he began to speak – this compressed his vocal cords. By changing the way he held his head and neck he found he could improve his breathing. This observation led to the Alexander technique.

If you habitually adopt postures that the body is not designed for, Alexander argued, your muscles and nerves are not going to work correctly. If your nerves do not work properly, neither do the organs they serve. So Alexander teachers (as practitioners are known) re-educate people about the correct postures. This restores the body's normal functions. As a result, the Alexander technique can benefit people with asthma.

A group of ten adults with asthma underwent 20 weekly Alexander technique lessons. They showed an improvement in their lung function: peak flow, for example, improved by nine per cent. The study's authors suggest that Alexander technique may increase the length of the torso because students are taught to stand upright. This increases muscle strength and enhances co-ordination. The difference is not huge – but it could make the difference between being on, say, step two and step three of the asthma management guidelines (page 137).

During an Alexander session, you will perform exercises to restore your bodily control, alleviate strain and relax. You will also learn to watch for and correct poor posture. Eventually, this becomes second nature. However, you cannot teach yourself the Alexander technique and teachers can take 30 or more sessions to re-educate your body. Alexander Technique International,★ the Alexander Teaching Network★ and the Society of Teachers of Alexander Technique★ all hold lists of approved teachers.

Herbalism

Asthma is mainly a disease of the affluent, developed world. Nevertheless, even people in rural parts of developing countries get asthma, so different cultures across the world have developed their own home-grown asthma treatments. The Chinese and Indians recognised lung diseases similar to asthma as long ago as 1550 BC: *Ma Huang* (also called ephedra), a herb containing a chemical related to the beta2-agonists (**Chapter 5**), was one of the first asthma treatments. People also smoked the leaves of the belladonna plant over 4,000 years ago to relieve symptoms.

During the early nineteenth century, asthmatics smoked thorn apple leaves. The active ingredient, stramonium, an anti-cholinergic (page 120), was the main ingredient in the popular Potter's Asthma Cure. Around the same time, people with asthma took belladonna's active ingredient – atropine, another anti-cholinergic – and drank strong coffee. We now know that coffee contains natural xanthines similar to theophylline (page 116). Indeed, drinking strong coffee can stave off very mild asthma symptoms. We have already seen that sodium cromoglycate (page 102) was derived from a plant product. In other words, traditional herbal remedies may have some basis in science. So can they be trusted?

Is herbalism safe?

Worldwide, about four billion people rely on plants as their main source of medicines. Herbalism is growing in popularity in the UK, and while no one seriously disputes its efficacy, some doctors question its safety. They point out that some herbs contain potent, even toxic, chemicals. Heroin, cocaine and cannabis are derived from plants, for example. And at high doses some plants – stramonium and atropine, for instance – are poisons. Herbalism's critics also argue that few herbal remedies undergo the same rigorous long-term safety testing as pharmaceutical drugs. When comfrey was tested by scientists, it was found to contain a chemical linked with liver damage in animals. The scientists injected only the purified chemical, at strengths humans would never use. However, the government now bans some comfrey preparations as a result.

Herbalists counter that they draw on a rich heritage. Herbalists know which herbs are dangerous and which are safe, and treat all plants with respect. Herbalists argue that you would have to eat about 5,500 comfrey leaves to reach the levels that were injected into animals in the experiment described above, pointing out that if the same rules applied to food the government should also have banned potatoes and peanuts: both contain potentially harmful chemicals. Furthermore, paracetamol and alcohol can cause liver damage, but are freely available.

Herbalism's critics also point out that herbal medicines can become contaminated. Some Asian herbal medicines may contain poisonous heavy metals such as lead, for example. And environmental factors, e.g. soil, climate and seasonal variants, can alter the subtle balance of active chemicals in herbs, known as the essential oil. However, reputable commercial manufacturers employ stringent quality control measures to minimise the risk of contamination and the balance of active chemicals is kept as consistent as possible.

Too much of anything can be harmful. Just because a product is natural does not mean it is safe. Indeed, some of the plants used to treat asthma – such as ephedra, lobelia and jasmine weed – should be used only by qualified medical herbalists. Other herbs used to treat asthma include grindelia, skunk cabbage, euphorbia, blood root, sundew and thyme. Herbal treatment may consist of tinctures (herbs in alcohol and water), syrups, teas, poultices or ointments. You may be asked to take an expectorant to clear the lungs of phlegm, and anti-spasmodics to reduce airway hyper-reactivity.

In moderation, herbalism appears to be a safe and effective complementary treatment for asthma and the stress caused by the condition. You should always consult a qualified herbalist. The Medicines Control Agency (MCA)★ is currently working with the British Herbal Medicine Association to formulate the correct protocol to ensure quality control and safety of all herbal products.

Chinese herbal medicine

Traditional Chinese medicine is one of the fastest-growing therapies in the West. Chinese herbalists believe that asthma and other illnesses are caused by a disruption in the flow of *qi* (pronounced 'chi'), or vital energy. This differs in everyone, so Chinese herbalists tailor the mix of herbs to the patient. The aim of treatment is to rebalance chi to restore the balance of energy in the body. You will probably be given a mixture of herbs and asked to prepare a *tang*, or soup, which you must drink several times a day.

Chinese medicine has had some remarkable successes – most notably in chronic eczema that did not respond to other treatments. As with herbal medicine, problems centre upon the difficulty of ensuring the quality of the herbs used. In addition, remedies might contain products from endangered species, such as tigers, rhinos or musk deer. To contact a qualified practitioner, contact the Register of Chinese Herbal Medicine.★

IMPORTANT

- Some herbs may interact with conventional medicines prescribed by your doctor, so you must tell your doctor if you are using herbal remedies and your herbalist needs to know which conventional drugs you are taking.
- Always consult a medical herbalist if you are pregnant or want to use herbs to treat a child. As with most drugs, it is probably prudent to avoid taking herbs during pregnancy. The National Institute of Medical Herbalists★ can help you find a local practitioner.

Homeopathy

Homeopathy is one of the most popular complementary therapies in the UK, although how it works is unclear. Some people find that it can alleviate asthma. Many scientists treat homeopathy's claims with scorn, despite a growing number of studies suggesting that it works. The problem with homeopathy is that it challenges the foundations of Western medicine.

Homeopathy's challenge to convention

The word homeopathy is derived from the Greek *homoios*, meaning 'like', and *pathos*, meaning 'suffering'. Homeopathy aims to work with the body by treating 'like with like'. For example, the bark of the cinchona tree alleviates symptoms in patients with malaria. But when healthy people take it, they develop symptoms similar to malaria. A number of other chemicals seem to share this property of causing symptoms in healthy people similar to those they treat. Homeopathic remedies kick-start the body into overcoming problems by itself. In contrast, conventional doctors aim to suppress symptoms – even though this can be counterproductive. For example, patients take aspirin for mild fever, but a raised temperature actually enhances the immune system's ability to fight infection.

By 1811, the German physician Dr Samuel Hahnemann was disillusioned. He had trained in orthodox medicine but his treatments often did more harm than good. Hahnemann believed that the symptoms of disease reflected the body's efforts to overcome

205

illness, in direct opposition to conventional doctors who believed illnesses caused the symptoms. Hahnemann abandoned his practice to experiment with other ways of healing.

Hahnemann experimented with single, uncompounded substances from plants, animals and minerals. To avoid side-effects, he diluted the substances in water and alcohol, which he mixed by vigorous shaking. Remarkably, Hahnemann found that the more dilute a substance became, the more potent its therapeutic action. However, substances that produced dissimilar symptoms to those being treated had no effect. Hahnemann called his method of diluting chemicals 'potentisation' and the serial dilutions 'potencies'. The dilution allows homeopaths to use poisons such as arsenic, morphine and cocaine safely to treat patients. Potentisation can also transform sand, salt and charcoal into potent remedies – as long as they are tailored for the right person suffering from the right disease.

Potentisation contributes to some doctors' accusations that homeopathy is biologically implausible. The formulations used are so dilute that the patient is unlikely to receive a single molecule of the 'active' ingredient. Moreover, the claim that a treatment becomes more potent as dilution increases goes against the fundamental principles of medical science. Pharmacologists propose that biologically active substances follow a 'dose–response' relationship: below a certain dose, a drug produces no effect. Above this threshold, response increases until it reaches a plateau, after which increasing the dose has no further effect. Homeopathy turns the dose–response relationship on its head. What makes the idea of homeopathy even more unpalatable for pharmacologists is that no one can adequately explain how it works.

Is homeopathy effective?

Homeopaths counter that the idea of like treating like is not as strange as it sounds. Vaccines work on much the same principle: doctors inject a small amount of either the whole, inactivated virus or a critical part of its protein coat. This triggers the same immune reaction as exposure to the live and virulent micro-organism would but does not cause serious symptoms. When you next encounter the organism your immune system is primed to tackle the infection rapidly. Other medical evidence would seem to support this theory – for example, hyperactive children can be treated with methylphenidate and amphetamine which are both powerful stimulants, and digitalis, used to treat heart failure, produces similar symptoms when taken in overdose quantities as those it treats.

Critics argue that the reported benefits of homeopathy could be due to a placebo effect. The power of the placebo is well recognised. Patients in trials of new medicines usually take either the drug or a tablet that looks and tastes identical, except that it lacks the active ingredient; neither patient or doctor knows if the treatment is active. The will to get better is very strong, and it is not unknown for patients to improve dramatically because they want to believe they are taking something that will cure them, even if this is not the case.

Homeopaths are holistic healers. Instead of enquiring only about symptoms, they will ask about your medical history, lifestyle, family history and even whether you are musical, scientific or artistic, sulky or rapidly angered, and so on. Homeopaths even note their clients' hair and eye colour and pay attention to their hopes and fears. In this way, they develop a detailed picture of the patient and match a remedy to this profile. Being paid so much attention might in itself make many people feel better. Cynics suggest that this intense interest shown to patients could increase the power of suggestion and enhance the potency of the placebo effect.

You might think that scientific studies would settle the question of the effectiveness of homeopathy. However, trials of homeopathy are extremely difficult to perform. Unlike drug studies, where a single medicine is prescribed to all patients, homeopathic treatment is individualised. No two patients have exactly the same personality, lifestyle or medical history, so people with different diseases may take the same homeopathic treatment, while people with the same disease could take different homeopathic remedies.

The few strictly controlled scientific studies that have been performed give homeopathy some credence.

- In 1986 a group of doctors from Glasgow compared the effects of a homeopathic preparation of grass seed pollen and a placebo in 144 hay fever sufferers. Neither the doctors nor the patients knew which they had received. Nevertheless, patients who received the homeopathic preparation reported fewer symptoms – and the doctors agreed.

- In 1994 the same doctors reported that homeopathy alleviated asthma more effectively than a placebo. Subjects who took the homeopathic preparation reported fewer and less intense symptoms – improvements persisted for eight weeks and lung function also improved. However, this result was relatively modest compared to the effect of modern anti-asthma medications.

- A summary of more than 100 studies investigating the effectiveness of homeopathy found that patients benefited in 77 trials.

Homeopathy is also successfully used to treat animals. It seems that the benefits of homeopathy cannot be dismissed as simply the placebo effect.

Using homeopathic remedies

Homeopathic tablets are chewed or sucked on an empty stomach. For rapid relief you may need to take tablets up to six times a day. In chronic ailments, the remedy is taken three times daily. Homeopaths subscribe to what they call the Rule of Twelve: that one month's treatment is needed for every year the person has had the disease. In other words, the rate of response is proportional to the duration of the disease.

Many people find that their symptoms initially get worse after starting homeopathic treatment. This is called 'aggravation reaction' and homeopaths regard it as a sign that the remedy is working. During this period, homeopaths suggest stopping the remedy and beginning again when the feeling passes. The Glasgow study of hay fever sufferers (see above) reported that patients who suffered an initial aggravation of symptoms improved.

This attitude towards symptoms marks a crucial difference in opinion between conventional and homeopathic practitioners. Many doctors regard an upsurge in symptoms as a reason to review treatment and possibly increase the dose until patients are either symptom-free or develop side-effects. In contrast, homeopathy does not suppress symptoms but claims to work with the body. After the initial worsening, your symptoms should start improving. If the improvement is maintained you can stop taking the tablets.

Finding a homeopath

Your GP can refer you to a homeopathic hospital or a local qualified homeopathy for treatment on the NHS. About 600 NHS doctors hold a postgraduate qualification in homeopathy and many more use some homeopathic remedies or refer patients for treatment. Some GPs are also qualified to provide homeopathic treatment either privately or on the NHS. The British Homeopathic Association★ can provide a list of medical homeopaths in your area.

The cynicism surrounding homeopathy may mean that your GP is reluctant to refer you. Many GPs do not realise, or choose to ignore, the extent of homeopathy's availability on the NHS. Theoretically, fundholding and the Patients' Charter should make referral easier, but you may have to stand your ground or consider a private consultation.

Some professional homeopaths are trained and practise but do not have medical qualifications. Make sure the therapist you choose is a member of the Society of Homeopaths,★ the professional body for homeopaths.

Hypnotherapy

For centuries, hypnotism was dismissed a stage trick, with its benefits confined to the gullible. In the late eighteenth century Franz Mesmer, a Viennese doctor, put large numbers of people into trances, calling the technique 'mesmerism'. His theatrical presentation alienated the medical community, however. Then towards the end of the last century the French physician Liébeault offered to treat people for free – provided they allowed him to hypnotise them. After putting his peasant volunteers into a hypnotic trance, Liébeault used hypnotism to suggest that their headaches, stomach aches and other pains would resolve. His success rate was high enough for his fame to spread. Liébeault is considered the founder of modern hynotherapy.

The technique was brought to the UK in the late nineteenth century by the Manchester surgeon James Braid, who coined the term hypnotism (from the Greek *hypnos*, meaning 'sleep'). Before the introduction of chloroform, major operations – including amputations and the removal of large tumours – were performed under hypnosis, apparently without patients experiencing pain. Although it was widely accepted among their Continental colleagues, the British medical profession refused to take hypnotism seriously.

However, the tide changed in the 1950s, when the *British Medical Journal* reported that hypnotism cured ichthyosis – a disfiguring disease where the skin appears rough and horny. A young boy was put into a hypnotic trance and told which areas of his skin would clear. These areas became almost normal. In 1955, hypnosis began to be accepted as a valid medical treatment for certain conditions. Most doctors now accept that hypnosis alleviates stress and helps patients quit smoking. However, it also seems that hypnosis may benefit people suffering from asthma.

For example, self-hypnosis can, if used promptly, alleviate asthma at the start of an attack. Sometimes the stress of a particular situation can trigger worsening symptoms – for instance, in one case a teenage girl had asthma only at weekends, when her father tended to drink excessively. Hypnosis can also help to alleviate stress that may trigger an attack. A year-long study underlined the benefits of hypnotherapy by showing that the symptoms of subjects who underwent hypnotism reduced by one-third. Another group who learnt simple relaxation techniques (see below) also benefited, but after eight months the patients who underwent hypnosis showed the best results.

Nevertheless, some doctors retain a lingering cynicism. Even today, a few scientists claim that subjects fake trances to please the hypnotist and audience. This may apply in some cases of stage hypnosis. However, it is hard to believe that a disfiguring skin disease would clear because the patient wanted to please the doctor.

The mystery of hypnotism

Not everyone is easily hypnotised. Even stage hypnotists pick their subjects carefully. For it to work, you have to *want* to be hypnotised. The best subjects tend to be people who immerse themselves in the imaginary worlds of books, films and plays and strongly identify with imaginary characters. Those who are motivated and keen to change their life are more likely to be easily hypnotised than people who like to be strongly in control or have conditions such as anorexia and obsessive compulsive disorder.

No one really understands how hypnotism works. It is clear that hypnotism is not a form of sleep. Most people feel tired, lethargic and drowsy during hypnosis. However, although the brain's electrical activity changes during a hypnotic trance the alterations do not resemble sleep. Indeed, electrical activity in the brain suggests the subject is fully awake during hypnosis. According to one favoured theory, the brain shuts off nerves supplying sensory information. This leaves subjects susceptible to certain suggestions. Another theory suggests that the left analytical side of the brain switches off, allowing the non-analytical right side of the brain to work. Certainly, during hypnosis subjects become very relaxed and less critical – which is why stage hypnotists can make people act as dogs or chickens.

For lists of qualified hypnotists contact the Central Register of Advanced Hypnotherapists★ or the National Register of Hypnotherapists and Psychotherapists.★

Meditation

Meditation can also alleviate asthma. Transcendental Meditation (TM),★ the best-studied form, was developed in 1960 by the Maharishi Mahesh Yogi. Many people find that TM reduces stress, and the link between asthma and the emotions is now well established. However, TM may also relax the muscles surrounding the bronchi and slow the respiration rate. In one study performed during the early 1970s, 21 patients kept diaries of their meditation habits, asthma symptoms, medication use and general wellbeing for six months. The doctors running the study also measured lung function.

- After three weeks of meditation, the subjects' asthma symptoms worsened, possibly because meditation made the practitioners more aware of their breathing. After this the symptoms began to improve.
- After six months patients reported fewer symptoms than before starting the experiment and showed improved lung function – the fall in bronchial resistance was particularly marked.
- Of the 18 patients who answered a questionnaire at the end of the study, 11 felt that TM helped their asthma. Another four felt that TM offered other benefits and continued to practise.

- The results were similar after another six months – a year from the start of the study. Some patients showed rather impressive improvements, and physicians also felt that patients benefited.

Though three of the five people who were on oral steroids at the start of the study were able to stop taking them, other patients tended to use the same amount of asthma medication. In other words, TM is an addition to, rather than a replacement for, anti-asthma drugs. This small study does, however, suggest that some people with asthma could benefit from meditation. Furthermore, the benefits are more than physical. Meditators often report an improvement in their academic performance, inter-personal relationships and sex life. Some studies even suggest that meditation boosts your IQ, increases creativity and sharpens the senses.

TM practitioners also tend to use fewer healthcare resources. Indeed, one major Dutch health insurance company offers reduced premiums to regular TM practitioners. However, meditators may be more likely to live otherwise healthy lives, which could mean they seek medical advice less often.

Learning meditation

People of all ages, backgrounds and religions meditate. In the UK 500–600 people learn TM each month (although 60 per cent give up doing it in the first year), and so far more than 150,000 people in the UK and over four million people worldwide have learnt the technique.

Classically, meditation involves sitting serenely on a mat with your eyes closed and your legs crossed, focussing on your breathing or a special saying (or *mantra*) for 20–30 minutes a couple of times a day. TM uses slightly shorter session of 15–20 minutes two or three times a day. While this may seem a considerable commitment of time in a busy life, meditators argue that taking 40–60 minutes a day to meditate helps you achieve more with less effort. After a while, meditation becomes part of your coping strategies that you call on when stressed – including at the start of an asthma attack.

How to meditate

To learn meditation correctly, you need instruction from a teacher.

However, you could get a feel for meditation by trying it for your-self, before investing time and money on a course.

- Find somewhere quiet. Beginners find meditation especially difficult where there are too many distractions.
- Sit comfortably. This doesn't need to be the full cross-legged 'lotus' position – a chair is fine. You'll need to sit still for about 20 minutes without the distractions of cramps and other aches.
- Now breathe deeply. Meditation teachers emphasise that most people tend to breathe into their chests instead of their abdomens, not using all the lungs. By concentrating, you can learn to breathe slowly and evenly in highly stressful situations – maybe even during an acute asthma attack.
- Now focus your attention. TM uses a *mantra* – a personal phrase or saying given to you by your teacher. But for this trial use a common *mantra* such as 'Om', or choose your own (it does not have to be exotic – any simple non-emotive word will do, even if it's nonsense). Other techniques encourage mind-ful meditation, where you maintain moment-to-moment awareness of the motion of your breath in and out of your nose and mouth. You can also focus on a candle flame, crystal or icon. These all have the same effect: they concentrate your mind and exclude distractions.
- Maintaining concentration for 20 minutes is far harder than it sounds. You will probably find your mind wanders off. Just accept these ramblings and re-focus your attention on the sub-ject. Try not to be annoyed with yourself.

Finding a teacher

TM★ is taught at 50 centres across the UK. If you decide TM is for you, you will probably go to four sessions on consecutive days and a further session three months later. TM has been studied the most and is the only form with a proven benefit in asthma, but it is not the only type of meditation. The Buddhist Society★ can put you in touch with teachers of traditional Buddhist or Zen medita-tion. More recently, Clinically Standardised Meditation was devel-oped by the psychologist Dr Patricia Carrington. You can learn this technique from tapes and books distributed by Learning for Life.★ Finally, meditation is an integral part of yoga. Contact The British Wheel of Yoga★ for further information.

Osteopathy

Osteopathy has a long heritage. Healers have used manipulation to treat spinal and back problems for over 2,000 years. Then in 1874 osteopathy's founder, the American physician Dr Andrew Taylor Still, developed a system of manipulation that alleviates a number of other disorders, including asthma. He coined the term osteopathy from the Greek *osteo* (meaning 'bone') and *pathos* (meaning 'disease'). Cranial osteopathy followed when, in the 1930s, doctors realised that bones making up the skull could move slightly. Cranial osteopaths very gently manipulate the bones in the skull to alter the movement of the body's tissue.

Osteopathy emphasises the importance of the interactions between the muscles, ligaments and the skeleton in maintaining health. Like many 'complementary' practitioners, Still believed in the body's innate ability to heal itself – provided the nerve and blood supply are uninterrupted. However, problems with the musculoskeletal system can block this healing process. So osteopaths use manipulation to realign structural deviations and abnormalities, including muscle spasms, spinal curvature and problems caused by poor posture.

Osteopathy, like the other methods in this section, reduces stress-related asthma triggers. Osteopaths can also stretch the diaphragm, make the soft cartilage in the thorax more flexible and improve posture. This, they claim, improves lung function and makes an asthma attack less likely.

Osteopaths begin by asking you to describe the factors that exacerbate and alleviate your asthma, so you might like to keep a diary for a couple of weeks before visiting your osteopath. He or she will also review your posture and the way you move and examine each vertebra for areas of tenderness, stiffness or abnormal shape.

Treatment includes manipulation, massage, rhythmic stretching and joint mobilisation. Osteopaths may stretch soft tissues, rhythmically move joints or apply a high velocity thrust to improve a joint's range of movement. These techniques aim to 'balance' the musculoskeletal system. As osteopathy aims to resolve the cause of your asthma, treatment may be applied some distance from your lungs. Furthermore, two patients with asthma suffering from apparently the same symptoms may be treated differently.

Usually osteopathy is not painful. You may feel tired, lightheaded and stiff, or ache for a couple of days afterwards. However, many people have no ill-effects at all and find osteopathy a good way to relax. Osteopathy aims to prevent the problem recurring. So osteopaths educate their clients about correct posture and emphasise the value of exercise in keeping the spine supple. They may also advise on diet.

Used improperly, osteopathy can do damage. You should always give your osteopath a full medical history as some conditions make osteopathy unsuitable. You can contact a registered practitioner through the Osteopathic Information Service,★ which represents osteopaths allied to a number of organisations.

Relaxation

Relaxation means more than curling up with a good book or watching your favourite television programme. As the mind and body are linked – you cannot be mentally tense and have a relaxed body and *vice versa* – relaxing the body relaxes the mind. Teenagers with psychogenic cough (page 69), for example, often benefit from learning relaxation techniques. Moreover, relaxation both helps reduce your risk of suffering an emotionally triggered attack and increases the likelihood that you will stay calm during an attack. Two of the most widely used techniques are progressive muscular relaxation and tension-relaxation.

Progressive muscular relaxation

Progressive muscle-relaxation often benefits those with asthma. In some studies, people are better able to cope with their symptoms and even show a small improvement in lung function, although other studies have not shown any benefit. While the direct effect on asthma symptoms remains an open question, there is no doubt that progressive muscle-relaxation helps everyone relax and cope with stress.

Progressive muscular relaxation aims to relax each part of your body in turn. Lie on the floor with a pillow under your head. After a few deep breaths, concentrate on your toes. Then say to yourself: 'My toes are tingling. They are becoming numb ...They are feeling heavier and heavier ...They are feeling increasingly relaxed ... the tension is draining away'. When your toes feel relaxed, move on to your calves.

Say to yourself: 'My calves are relaxed ... They are feeling softer and heavier ... They are feeling numb and more relaxed ... the tension is draining away'. Once your calves are relaxed, move on to your thighs. Work through the rest of your body in an upwards direction (hands, arms, torso, shoulders, face) – once you have worked to your forehead, lie still for a few minutes before standing up.

Tension-relaxation

When you employ tension-relaxation, you tense a muscle for about ten seconds before relaxing. As with progressive muscular relaxation, the whole body is involved. Each exercise of the relevant part is repeated three times, slowly, gently and gradually. You repeat the set twice, making nine repetitions of the tension-relaxation for each group of muscles. After this you rest for 20–30 minutes. Most teachers advise mastering one muscle group at a time, so it could take two or three months before you can tense and relax your whole body.

You should lie on the floor with a pillow under your head, or sit in a chair that supports your back. As an example, put your hands by your side. Now clench your fists as hard as you can. Hold the fists for ten seconds. Now slowly relax your fists and let your hands hang loosely by your side. When focussing on your shoulders, shrug them as high as possible; when concentrating on the back, arch your back as high as you can, leaving only your head and buttocks touching the chair or floor. Tense your muscles when you inhale. During the tension do not hold your breath, but breathe slowly and rhythmically. Then exhale as you relax.

After practising tension-relaxation exercises for a few months, you will come to recognise when your muscles are tense. Most of us live for years with considerable muscle tension, so our bodies become used to a certain level. But this means that we cannot gauge the true state of our muscles. Tension-relaxation exercises familiarise us with our muscles.

IMPORTANT

If you suffer from back problems you should talk to your doctor or physiotherapist before performing tension-relaxation exercises.

Relaxation's golden rules

Whichever technique you choose, following a few simple rules will help you make the most of your relaxation sessions.

- Try to relax every day. The best time is first thing in the morning: the house tends to be quieter and interruptions are less likely. Try setting your alarm half-an-hour earlier.
- Avoid relaxation exercises last thing at night – you will probably not be able to concentrate as well and you could fall asleep rather than relax.
- Shut your eyes.
- Take the phone off the hook or put on the answerphone.
- Do not relax on a full stomach. After a meal, blood diverts from your muscles to your stomach – trying to relax tense muscles on a full stomach can cause cramps. As relaxation exercises increase your awareness of your body's functions, a full stomach can be a distraction.
- Find a quiet room where you can sit in a comfortable chair that supports your back, or lie down – you may want to put cushions under your neck and knees.
- Make yourself comfortable. Take your shoes off and wear loose-fitting clothes, switch off any bright lights and make sure the room temperature is not too hot or too cold.
- Play a favourite piece of music, not too loud. Many people find music helps them relax and minimises interruptions. You could try classical music or one of the growing number of 'New Age' and ambient tapes and CDs.
- Be passive: don't start worrying about whether you are relaxed enough.
- Concentrate on your breathing. Most of us breathe shallowly, using the upper parts of our lungs. However, to relax you need to breathe deeply and slowly without gasping. Put one hand on your chest and the other on your abdomen. Breathe normally. You may find – especially if you are tense – that the hand on your chest moves, while the hand on the abdomen remains almost still. The hand on your stomach should rise and fall while the one on your chest hardly alters. Focussing on your breathing may improve your perception of lung function and symptoms but is unlikely to replace a peak flow meter.

THE WHICH? GUIDE TO MANAGING ASTHMA

- Don't give up. Some days you will find it easier to relax than others. After a while, relaxation sessions will become part of your everyday life. You just have to give them a chance.

Yoga

Yoga was first practised in some form 5,000 years ago in India. It reached Britain during the Victorian era, but did not become popular until the 1960s. Today, yoga brings millions of people around the world inner peace, relief from stress and improved health. It may also benefit asthma. A study found that young people with asthma who practised yoga enjoyed improved lung function and exercise capacity compared to those who did not take it up. Furthermore, over two years the yoga practitioners used fewer asthma drugs and experienced fewer symptoms.

Yoga brings other benefits as well. It keeps your mind and body supple and relaxes and strengthens stressed-out physiques. In other words, Yoga is far removed from the image of forcing your body into strange positions in a draughty church hall. Yoga is a complete system that helps you manage your life.

In common with most other complementary therapies, yoga conceives of all aspects of your life – consciousness, mind, energy and body – as intertwined. Yoga aims to harmonise these aspects: the Sanskrit root of the word yoga means 'to unite'. Yoga seeks to achieve this unity in three ways.

Posture

Yoga is perhaps best known for the postures that improve our control of our unruly bodies. Known as *asanas*, these postures are more than physical exercises. Correctly performed, *asanas* involve mental control, correct breathing – which may help asthma – and using your body with minimum effort and tension. The postures gently stretch and contract muscles and joints. This allows you to move more freely and improves stamina, flexibility and strength. There are some 80 postures, though most people only use 20. Teachers claim that *asanas* train the mind and raise consciousness.

Mental balance

Yoga practitioners assert that a raised consciousness promotes positive and stimulating effects. For example, Yoga bolsters your stress defences and may help reduce your fears about future asthma attacks. We worry about many events that have not happened yet – and probably never will – instead of devoting our energy to the present. Yoga and meditation help practitioners live in the present.

Breath control

Like many other complementary medicines, yoga emphasises correct breathing. When you are tense, your breaths tend to be shallow and centre on the upper chest. This is not advisable if you are healthy and even less so if your lung function is already compromised because of asthma. By performing breathing exercises – *pranayama* – that restrain and control the breath, yoga practitioners learn to use the entire lung. These exercises may benefit patients with asthma and other respiratory disorders. By practising yoga, you will become more aware of your lungs and how they feel. This may mean that you are more likely to be able to detect a change in your symptoms (not accurately perceived by some people with asthma). This is not a substitute for your peak flow meter, however.

Yoga practitioners believe that breath control allows them to regulate their physical and mental processes and helps them attain the ultimate goal of yoga – self-enlightenment.

Finding a yoga class

You should perform yoga in a quiet, warm, well-ventilated room. Wear comfortable, light clothes and do not practise on a full stomach. You will need to attend classes to learn yoga correctly. Apart from this you must be prepared to set aside some time to practise each day – ideally 20–30 minutes. Be prepared not to see instant benefits. It takes time to learn how to train your body.

A wide range of books and videos can provide you with a basic understanding of yoga and its benefits. However, you should learn yoga from a teacher. The British Wheel of Yoga★ can provide further details. The Yoga for Health Foundation★ runs yoga retreats. Your library or adult education centre may also have details of local courses.

CHAPTER 10

TOWARDS A CURE

ASTHMA treatment has undoubtedly improved dramatically over the last few years. Despite an ever-increasing number of people with asthma, the death rate shows encouraging signs of beginning to fall. More importantly, modern drugs mean that most people with asthma can lead normal lives. They can even take part in the Olympics, win gold medals and break world records.

However, new asthma treatments are still needed. For example, treating children under two years of age remains difficult. Bronchodilator and anti-inflammatory syrups that do not cause side-effects would make life much easier for parents. Moreover, many people dislike taking treatments for life, despite reassurances about the safety of their drugs. Today's delivery devices are often difficult to use – many patients prefer tablets to inhalers. And there remains a small proportion of patients with severe asthma who fail to respond adequately to any inhaled therapy. They may require regular and prolonged courses of oral steroids – with all the associated risks of side-effects (**Chapter 5**). Fortunately, several new asthma treatments are on the horizon. Furthermore, doctors are devising new ways of diagnosing asthma.

Both of these developments are driven by doctors' increasing understanding of the inflammation underlying asthma. As we saw in **Chapter 1**, inflammation in the lungs is orchestrated and co-ordinated by a vast array of chemical messengers. Pharmacologists – scientists who develop new drugs – are testing the suitability of chemicals that target these mediators to become new anti-asthma medicines. Yet this targeted approach raises a fundamental question: can human ingenuity outwit the immune system?

The search for new asthma drugs

In 1938, scientists injected cobra venom into the lung of a guinea pig. At that time, histamine was believed to be responsible for various allergic reactions, and to cause the bronchoconstriction characteristic of asthma. But when anti-histamines were given to the animal, they did not inhibit the venom's effect. This suggested that some other substance was responsible. Later studies showed that other antigens also triggered the release of the same mystery substance, which scientists christened 'slow-reacting substance of anaphylaxis'. It was not until 1979 that researchers finally discovered that the slow-reacting substance of anaphylaxis was a cocktail of three leukotrienes, known as C4, D4 and E4. We now know that these are part of a large family of leukotrienes that are proving tempting targets for pharmacologists trying to develop new treatments for asthma.

Zafirlukast (page 103), the first drug to target the leukotrienes, was launched recently and is currently being assessed in children aged under 12 years of age. Over the next few years, a number of other drugs that work by blocking the action of this key inflammatory mediator are likely to be launched. Some – for example, a drug called zileuton – reduce leukotriene formation. Others, like zafirlukast, blocks leukotriene's action by binding to its receptor site – acting as an antagonist (page 108).

Montelukast (Singulair), for example, is a potent new leukotriene receptor antagonist. In a recent study, 68 patients took a tablet containing either montelukast or placebo once daily. FEV1 (page 76) improved by 13 per cent in patients taking montelukast compared to a four per cent improvement among those receiving inactive placebo. Furthermore:

- daytime symptoms and 'rescue' beta-agonist use fell by 24 per cent
- nocturnal awakenings and exacerbations both fell by 31 per cent
- patients experienced more days free of asthma – a 37 per cent improvement.

There was little difference in side-effects between the inactive placebo and montelukast.

Another approach targets thromboxane, an inflammatory mediator that seems to be especially important in bronchial hypersensitivity, or twitchy airways. Pharmacologists are now developing drugs that block thromboxane production. One of the first of these was recently introduced in Japan. Europe will probably not be too far behind.

Pharmacologists are also investigating drugs related to theophylline (page 116), which is undergoing a renaissance as doctors increasingly recognise its ability to dampen the inflammation underlying asthma. Pharmacologists are currently seeking to fine-tune this effect. Theophylline acts partly by blocking an enzyme called phosphodiesterase that helps convey messages *inside* the cell – a crucial difference between drugs that work in this way and medicines that block the effect of mediators *before* they bind to receptors on the cell surface. Different cells express different types of phosphodiesterase (PDE). So, for example, many of the cells involved in inflammation in asthma express a subtype of this enzyme (PDE4). Several drugs that block phosphodiesterase 4 are now being developed and should become available over the next few years.

Is the new generation of drugs better?
While drugs acting on the leukotrienes and phosphodiesterase show some promise, the benefits and safety of the agents in development remain to be established in large-scale clinical studies. They have the advantage of being effective oral anti-inflammatories that could make the problem of poor inhaler technique redundant. Yet whether they offer any other additional advantages over inhaled steroids remains to be seen.

Other developments

Another approach in the fight against asthma is to block the allergy antibody's binding site on mast cells. As noted in **Chapter 1**, specific IgE antibodies bind to mast cells, triggering the release of histamine and other inflammatory mediators and causing the symptoms of asthma. Scientists are developing chemicals that 'sit' on the binding site and prevent the antibody from anchoring there. Clinical trials of these 'IgE antagonists' could begin in the next couple of years.

Other scientists are applying advances made in other areas of medicine. For example, cyclosporin A is the drug largely responsible for making kidney transplants almost routine. It prevents the immune system from recognising that the transplanted kidney is foreign tissue and rejecting it. While cyclosporin A is widely used in transplant medicine, it causes a number of side-effects when taken orally, so it is used in experimental studies only among people with very severe asthma who are not responding adequately to oral steroids. In early studies about half of these patients, who were taking an average of 30mg prednisolone daily, were able to reduce their dose to 11mg a day. One way to limit the side-effects may be to develop an inhaled formulation of cyclosporin A – in the same way that inhaled steroids reduce the risk of side-effects seen with oral steroids.

Many other agents are being developed to reduce further the likelihood of a patient rejecting a transplanted organ: some of these are being assessed in severe asthma. These agents may, by suppressing the lung's immunity, increase patients' likelihood of contracting severe respiratory infections – or even cancer. Nevertheless, these powerful immunosuppressants may find a role in the treatment of people with severe asthma. As our knowledge of them evolves, they provide scientists with leads on how to bring about a chemical change in the molecule to provide safer treatment.

Foiling the immune system

The current trend towards using drugs targeting a single mediator in the immune response leads to a fundamental question – can we develop medicines able to foil the immune system?

Steroids (see **Chapter 5**) suppress the entire immune response – they are 'non-specific'. Nedocromil (page 101) and sodium cromoglycate (page 102) inhibit a key cell, the mast cell. By contrast, zafirlukast inhibits just one specific type of leukotriene, only one of 20 or so mediators implicated in asthmatic inflammation. Doctors do not yet know which of the immune mediators are responsible for the particular symptoms of asthma, although they have their suspicions: leukotrienes may be important in exercise-induced asthma, for example. Despite taking such a selective approach, zafirlukast nonetheless appears to be effective.

However, some previous specifically targeted drugs that showed promise in animal experiments failed when they reached the clinic, including drugs blocking platelet activating factor (PAF). PAF is a potent trigger of inflammation. In animals and in humans under-going inhalation challenge tests (page 79), it triggers profound bronchoconstriction and airway hyper-reactivity, also recruiting other white blood cells into the area of inflammation. It seemed a tempting target for drug development: block PAF, pharmacologists thought, and you'll block asthma. Yet though a number of PAF antagonists have been developed, none seems to have any effect on either the early or late phase of an asthma attack (pages 21–2).

In some ways, we are trying to outwit evolution. We would not survive very long without an immune system, so the human race evolved 'back-up' systems in case anything went wrong. A particu-lar immune response may therefore be triggered by several differ-ent mediators – another taking over if the usual mediator is blocked. This is known as 'redundancy'. In other words, blocking a single mediator may not prevent asthma. The immune system may simply recruit other mediators to perform the task of the blocked messenger.

This does not seem to occur with zafirlukast. However, it may partly explain why the early promise of PAF antagonists was not realised. As a result, a number of companies are exploring the pos-sibility of developing new, non-specific inhaled steroids as well as specific drugs, and improving delivery devices.

The wider picture

In addition to developing new treatments, researchers are also try-ing to enhance the amount of medication that reaches your lungs and improve diagnosis.

A number of new inhalers are likely to be launched over the next few years as the world-wide CFC ban begins to bite (page 129). Researchers are also formulating more effective ways to deliver drugs to the lung. For example, the long-acting bron-chodilator eformoterol (page 115) formulated as a Turbohaler was recently approved in Sweden and should be launched in the UK during 1997.

Doctors have yet to devise an unequivocal diagnostic procedure for asthma, as explained in **Chapter 4**. We clearly need more accu-rate, sensitive and reliable diagnostic tests. As a result, new tests are being developed that should help doctors gain a better insight into the severity of the underlying inflammation. For example, these new tests – which measure levels of some of the key inflammatory mediators in asthma – could help determine whether a positive skin test is clinically relevant to the true cause of a patient's asthma. (Skin tests can show whether someone is allergic to a trigger, but not if the allergen is capable of causing an asthma attack.) The tests could also guide therapy – a more intense inflammation will produce higher levels of mediators and may require more intensive anti-inflammatory treatment, for example. Finally, doctors will be able to monitor the effectiveness of therapy.

Eosinophil cationic protein (ECP) is currently the leading contender for this new test. ECP is secreted by eosinophils, one of the white blood cells controlling the inflammation underlying asthma. Studies so far suggest that measuring blood levels of ECP may hold some promise of reflecting how severe the asthma is, allowing doctors to monitor progress and the response to anti-inflammatory treatment. For example, ECP levels rise if the allergen load increases and declines once steroids begin to work. However, measurements of ECP have not been shown to reflect the severity of the asthma and further studies are needed before the test becomes part of routine clinical practice.

Other studies are providing new insights into the biology of asthma. For example, recent studies examined the beta2-receptors in the lung and found that not all were equal. Differences in the genetic make-up of individuals subtly alter the structure of the beta2-receptor. The less common variations may influence a patient's response to drugs – rendering beta2-agonists (page 107) less effective – and increase the risk that he or she will develop severe asthma. Genetic tests that look for variants in the beta2-receptor may allow doctors to assess the severity of a person's asthma before treatment and help in the formulation of a management plan.

Furthermore, a study from Southampton found that 39 per cent of children with at least one atopic parent who tested positive on a skin test for milk allergen wheezed at the age of two years. Forty per cent developed eczema. This raises the prospect that doctors may be able to predict which children are likely to develop allergic diseases and devise preventative strategies. However, only 14 per cent of the children who developed eczema or wheezed tested positive to milk allergen. So there is some way to go before doctors can predict with any degree of accuracy which children will develop asthma.

New hope for people with asthma

Another approach aims to prevent asthma from developing in the first place. Allergic (atopic) eczema is often the first sign that a child is susceptible to asthma. For example, between 3 and 11 per cent of children develop atopic eczema during the first year of life. About half of these go on to develop asthma.

A study known as ETAC (Early Treatment of the Atopic Child) is now underway in 56 hospitals across Europe and Canada. It aims to find out whether treating children with cetirizine (Zirtek) – a drug which combines antihistamine and anti-inflammatory actions – delays or prevents the progression of atopic eczema into asthma. Results will not available until the end of 1997 or early 1998. ETAC is also assessing the role of biological markers such as eosinophil cationic protein (above) to see if they can be used to help identify those children likely to develop asthma.

It is also possible that doctors may be able to vaccinate people against asthma. Researchers in Nottingham have developed a genetically engineered enzyme produced by the house dust mite. Modifying the enzyme could form the basis of a vaccine. However, it will be several years before human trials begin.

In the meantime, human trials have already begun investigating another promising candidate vaccine. The study included 13 patients who were allergic to foods. After being vaccinated they were challenged with the trigger that affected them. None of the patients developed an allergic reaction. Furthermore, the vaccine prevented anaphylactic shock in two people – one of whom was sensitive to nuts, the other to fish. It is early days, however, and many more people will need to receive the vaccine before doctors can be sure that it is effective and safe. If the early promise is fulfilled, the vaccine will be offered first to adults with severe asthma. Children will follow only after extensive further testing. But these studies raise the intriguing possibility that asthma may eventually be cured.

Gene therapy may offer another possible cure for asthma. As noted in **Chapter 2**, genetic factors play an important role in asthma and other allergic diseases. Gene therapy aims to replace a defective gene with a healthy one, although its major problem is how to get the healthy gene into the cell. Fortunately, nature has provided the ideal carrier. Viruses cause disease by 'hijacking' the genetic machinery of cells and making the genes create new viral particles rather than sustain a patient's health and well-being. Scientists are consequently using genetic engineering to place healthy genes inside a virus that has its replication genes 'switched off'. As a result, the virus inserts the healthy gene into the patient's genetic machinery but cannot replicate. Though some – but by no means all – scientists regard the results so far as disappointing, gene therapy is being assessed in cystic fibrosis and certain cancers.

There are problems specific to asthma. Unlike cystic fibrosis, caused by a single defect, asthma is due to a number of genetic defects on at least three of the body's 23 pairs of chromosomes. Furthermore, not everyone who inherits the atopy gene reacts in the same way. The environment is just as important as your genetic make-up. Again, this marks a difference to cystic fibrosis, which you will develop irrespective of the environment if you carry the genes (although the severity varies).

As a result, experiments using gene therapy will have to be stayed until scientists better understand the cause of asthma. Gene therapy is unlikely ever to become a widely used treatment for asthma – its expense could be prohibitive and there are some concerns over its safety. However, gene therapy does offer the prospect of curing asthma, especially in severely ill people who do not respond to other therapies.

In the meantime, inhaled steroids will remain the mainstay of asthma treatment. Effective treatments are now available for most people who have asthma, and in some ways the real challenge is not developing new treatments but ensuring that we make the most of drugs already at doctors' disposal as well as using the self-help measures described in earlier chapters. Hopefully, by following the advice in this book you can control your asthma – rather than letting it control you.

GLOSSARY

Acaricides House dust mites are one of the commonest allergens among people with asthma. Acaricides kill the house dust mite.

Allergen A substance that triggers an allergic reaction.

Allergy Allergy develops when an oversensitive immune system reacts strongly to a substance that most people find benign. Allergies can develop in the skin (eczema), lungs (asthma) or upper respiratory tract and eyes (allergic rhinitis – hay fever).

Anaphylaxis A severe, potentially life-threatening, allergic reaction.

Antibodies Proteins circulating in the blood that attach to allergens and stimulate the immune system.

Antigens Foreign substances, usually proteins, that trigger an immune response.

Antihistamine A drug that antagonises – blocks – histamine.

Anti-inflammatories Drugs that reduce the immune response and dampen down inflammation.

Asthma Asthma – chronic inflammation of the airways – leaves bronchi hyper-responsive so that they narrow readily when exposed to a wide range of triggers. As a result, patients cough, wheeze and complain of chest tightness and breathlessness.

Atopy A genetic propensity to develop allergic conditions.

B lymphocytes White blood cells, formed in the bone marrow, that mature into plasma cells. B lymphocytes produce antibodies and protect the body from invasion by foreign proteins.

Beta2-agonists Drugs that bind to beta-receptors in the muscle surrounding the bronchi, leading to relaxation. Beta2-agonists are bronchodilators.

Bronchi The numerous small airways in the lung that become inflamed in asthma.

Bronchoconstriction Contraction of the muscle surrounding the bronchi, leading to narrowing of the airways.

Bronchodilators Drugs, such as the beta2-agonists, that open the bronchi.

Compliance The ability to follow the doctor's instructions (usually with reference to drugs).

Corticosteroids Corticosteroids reduce the immune response and dampen inflammation.

Cross-sensitive Many people allergic to one allergen also react to another. So people with food allergies often cross-react to several different foods.

Dander Small pieces of fur and skin shed by animals.

Diurnal variation The natural changes in airway calibre during the day. The airways tend to be narrowest at night.

Dyspnoea Laboured breathing.

Eosinophil White blood cells that protect the body from parasitic infections. Circulating eosinophil levels increase in patients with asthma.

Exacerbation A worsening of asthma symptoms.

FEV1 Forced expiratory volume in one second – a measure of lung function.

FVC The maximum volume of air expelled after a full breath in – a measure of lung function.

Histamine An inflammatory mediator released from mast cells, histamine stimulates mucus production and contracts smooth muscle. It also allows blood and fluid to leak into tissue, producing redness and swelling.

Immune response The reaction of the body's defences (the immune system) to an invading organism or infection.

Immunoglobulins A family of proteins that act as antibodies. There are six main classes, each of which triggers a different aspect of the immune response. IgE, for example, protects the body from parasitic infections. People with asthma produce high levels of IgE in response to allergens.

Immunotherapy Patients undergoing immunotherapy are injected with increasing amounts of allergen, which, for reasons no-one understands, may alleviate allergic disorders.

Inflammation A local protective response following injury.

Inflammatory mediators Chemicals that co-ordinate the immune response.

Leukotrienes A type of inflammatory mediator.

Macrophages A group of white blood cells that digest cell debris and foreign particles. Macrophages also digest allergens and present the fragments to T lymphocytes.

Mast cells Each allergen molecule cross-links two IgE molecules on the surface of the mast cell. As a result, the mast cell releases a cocktail of inflammatory mediators, including histamine.

NSAIDS (non-steroidal anti-inflammatory drugs) A group of drugs, which includes aspirin and ibuprofen, widely used to treat mild pain and inflammatory diseases such as arthritis. In some people with asthma, NSAIDs or related natural chemicals called salicylates may provoke an attack.

Peak expiratory flow rate See peak flow.

Peak flow The maximum flow rate of air breathed out – the most widely used measure of lung function.

Plasma cells Mature B lymphocytes that secrete antibodies.

Preventer See anti-inflammatories.

Reliever See bronchodilators.

Rhinitis Nasal inflammation.

Salicylates See NSAIDS.

Sensitiser An irritant that leaves the patient's lung sensitive to that, and occasionally other, chemical(s) or allergen(s).

Skin prick test A solution of a suspected allergen is dropped onto the skin. Each drop is then pricked with a needle. A red weal that develops within 10–20 minutes suggests that the patient may be sensitive to that allergen.

Steroids See corticosteroids.

T lymphocytes White blood cells, produced in the thymus gland, that co-ordinate the immune response. There are two broad classes of T lymphocyte: killer T cells and helper T cells. Killer T cells, as their name suggests, destroy invading bacteria and viruses. Helper T cells stimulate B lymphocytes to develop into plasma cells.

Upper respiratory tract The nose, mouth, trachea and larynx.

ADDRESSES

Action on Smoking and Health (ASH)
16 Fitzhardinge Street,
London W1H 9PL
0171-224 0743

Alexander Teaching Network
PO Box 53,
Kendal, Cumbria LA9 4UP

Alexander Technique International
142 Thorpedale Road,
London N4 3BS
0171-281 7639

Anaphylaxis Campaign
PO Box 149,
Fleet, Hampshire GU13 9XU
(01252) 318723

Arthritis Care
18 Stephenson Way,
London NW1 2HD
0171-916 1500

Arthritis & Rheumatism Council for Research (ARC)
PO Box 177,
Chesterfield, Derbyshire
S41 7TQ
(01246) 558033
send sae for publications list and free booklet

British Acupuncture Council
Park House,
206-208 Latimer Road,
London W10 6RE
0181-964 0222

British Allergy Foundation
0181-303 8583 (*helpline*)

British Association for Counselling (BAC)
1 Regent Place,
Rugby, Warwickshire CV21 2PJ
(01788) 578328

British Complementary Medicine Association
249 Fosse Road South,
Leicester LE3 1AE
0116-282 5511

British Homeopathic Association
27A Devonshire Street,
London W1N 1RJ
0171-935 2163

British Lung Foundation
78 Hatton Garden,
London EC1N 8JR
0171-831 5831

British Wheel of Yoga
1 Hamilton Place,
Boston Road, Sleaford,
Lincolnshire NG34 7ES
(01529) 306851

The Buddhist Society
58 Eccleston Square,
London SW1V 1PH
0171-834 5858

Central Register of Advanced Hypnotherapists
28 Finsbury Park Road,
London N4 2JX
0171-359 6991

Chest, Heart and Stroke Scotland
65 North Castle Street,
Edinburgh EH2 3LT
0131-225 6963
(0345) 720720 (*helpline 9.30-12.30, 1.30-4 Mon-Fri*)

Council for Complementary and Alternative Medicine
Park House,
206-208 Latimer Road,
London W10 6RE
0181-968 3862

Ethics and Anti-doping Directorate of the UK Sports Council
0171-380 8030

Greenpeace
Canonbury Villas,
London N1 2PN
0171-865 8183
http://www.greenpeace.org.uk

Friends of the Earth
56-58 Alma Street,
Luton, Bedfordshire LU1 2PH
(01582) 482297
http://www.foe.co.uk/

Health and Safety Executive
(0541) 545500 (*information line*)
or check phone book for your local office

Institute for Complementary Medicine
PO Box 194,
London SE16 1QZ
0171-237 5165

Learning for Life
The Coach House,
Chinewood Manor,
32 Manor Road, Bournemouth,
Dorset BH1 3EZ
(01202) 390008

Medic Alert Foundation
1 Bridge Wharf,
156 Caledonian Road,
London N1 9UU
0171-833 3034
(0800) 581420 (*freephone*)

Medicines Control Agency (MCA)
1 Nine Elms Lane,
London SW8 5NQ
0171-273 0000

National Asthma Campaign
Providence House,
Providence Place,
London N1 0NT
(0345) 010203 (*helpline*)
0171-971 0444 (*information and
May-August pollen line*)
0171-226 2260 (*office*)

National Eczema Society
163 Eversholt Street,
London NW1 1BU
0171-388 4097

**National Institute of Medical
Herbalists**
56 Longbrook Street,
Exeter, Devon EX4 6AH
(01392) 426022

National Osteoporosis Society
PO Box 10,
Radstock, Bath,
N.E. Somerset BA3 3YB
(01761) 471771 (*helpline*)

**National Register of
Hypnotherapists and
Psychotherapists**
12 Cross Street, Nelson,
Lancashire BB9 7EN
(01282) 699378

Osteopathic Information Service
PO Box 2074,
Reading, Berkshire RG1 4YR
(01734) 512051

Quitline
Victory House,
170 Tottenham Court Road,
London W1P 0HA
(0800) 002200 (*freephone*)

**Register of Chinese Herbal
Medicine**
PO Box 400,
Wembley HA9 9NZ
0181-904 1357 (*answerphone*)

Society of Homeopaths
2 Artizan Road, Northampton
NN1 4HU
(01604) 21400

**Society of Teachers of the
Alexander Technique**
20 London House,
266 Fulham Road,
London SW10 9EL
0171-351 0828

Transcendental Meditation (TM)
Freepost,
London SW1P 4YY
(0990) 143733

Yoga for Health Foundation
Ickwell Bury, Ickwell Green,
Biggleswade, Bedfordshire
SG18 9EF
(01767) 627271

BIBLIOGRAPHY

Books

Atherton, D.J. 1995. *Eczema in childhood: the facts*. Oxford

Barnes, P.J. and Levy, J. 1984. *Nocturnal asthma*. RSM

Dorfman, W. and Cristofar, L. 1985. *Psychosomatic illness review*. Macmillan

Gary, J. 1986. *Food intolerance: fact & fiction*. Grafton

Greener, M. 1996. *The Which? guide to managing stress*. Which? Books

Hafen, B. and Frandsen, K. 1984. *An A-Z of alternative medicine*. Sheldon Press

Macdonald, A. 1982. *Acupuncture from ancient art to modern medicine*. George Allen & Unwin

Mills, S.Y. 1993. *The A-Z of modern herbalism*. Paragon

Morgan, W.K.C. and Seaton, A. 1996. *Occupational lung disease* (3e). WB Saunders

Nightingale, M. 1987. *Acupuncture*. Optima

Rowlands, B. 1997. *The Which? guide to complementary medicine*. Which? Books

Small, R. and Johnson, M. (ed) 1995. *Beta-adrenoceptor agonists and the airways*. RSM

Waxman, D. 1981. *Hypnosis: a guide for patients and practitioners*. George Allen & Unwin

British Guidelines on Asthma Management

The guidelines are published in the February 1997 supplement to *Thorax* (**52**, suppl. 1)

Selected Papers

Barnes, P.J. Immunomodulation as asthma therapy: where do we stand? *European Respiratory Journal*, **9** (suppl. 22), 154–159

Barnes, P.J. Inhaled glucocorticoids: new developments relevant to updating of the asthma management guidelines. *Respiratory Medicine*, **90**, 379–84

Beasley, R., Burgess, C., Crane, J. *et al*. A review of the studies of the asthma mortality epidemic in New Zealand. *Allergy Proceedings*, **16**, 27–32

Bindslev-Jensen, C., Skov, P.S., Madsen, F. *et al*. Food allergy and food intolerance – what is the difference? *Annals of Allergy*, **72**, 317–20

Boorsma, M., Andersson, N., Larsson, P. *et al*. Assessment of the relative systemic potency of inhaled fluticasone and budesonide. *European Respiratory Journal*, **9**, 1427–32

Brugman, S.M. and Larsen, G.L. Asthma in infants and small children. *Clinics in Chest Medicine*, **16**, 637–56

Bush, R.K. and Hefle, S.L. Lessons and myths regarding cross-reacting foods *Allergy Proceedings*, **16**, 245–6

Chilmonczyk, B.A., Salmun, L.M., Megathlin, K.N. *et al*. Association between exposure to environmental tobacco smoke and exacerbations of asthma in children. *New England Medical Journal*, **328**, 1665–9

Clark, D.J., Clark, R.A. and Lipworth, B.J. Adrenal suppression with inhaled budesonide and fluticasone propionate given by large volume spacer to asthmatic children. *Thorax*, **51**, 941–43

de Jong, J.W., Postma, D.S., de Monchy, J.G.R. *et al*. A review of nedocromil sodium in asthma therapy. *European Respiratory Review*, **3**, 511–19

Fireman, P. Beta2 agonists and their safety in the treatment of asthma. *Allergy Proceedings*, **16**, 235–9

Frew, A.J. Conventional and alternative allergen immunotherapy: do they work? Are they safe? *Clinical and Experimental Allergy*, **24**, 416–22

Gern, J.E., Schroth, M.K. and Lemanske, P.F. Childhood asthma: older children and adolescents. *Clinics in Chest Medicine*, **16**, 657–70

Greener, M. Do inhaled steroids inhibit childhood growth? *Paediatrics Today*, September 1996

Greener, M. Asthma – beyond steroids. *Pharmaceutical Times*, May 1997, 22–4

Greener, M. Asthma: treating more than the lungs. *Practice Nursing*, **7**, 19–23

Harding, S.M. The human pharmacology of fluticasone propionate. *Respiratory Medicine*, **84** (suppl. A), 25–9

Hopkin, J.M. Genetics of atopy. *Pediatric Allergy and Immunology*, **6**, 139–44

Johnson, M. Pharmacodynamics and pharmacokinetics of inhaled glucocorticoids. *Journal of Allergy and Clinical Immunology*, **97**, 169–76

Johnson, M. Pharmacology of long-acting beta-agonists. *Annals of Allergy, Asthma, and Immunology*, **74**, 177–9

Kamada, A.K. and Szefler, S.J. Glucocorticoids and growth in asthmatic children. *Pediatric Allergy and Immunology*, **6**, 145–54

Kowalski, M.L. Aspirin-sensitive rhinosinusitis/asthma syndrome – pathophysiology and management. *ACI International*, **8**, 49–57

McFadden, E.R. and Gilbert, I.A. Exercise-induced asthma. *New England Journal of Medicine*, **330**, 1362–7

O'Byrne, P.M. What is asthma? An update on the mechanisms. *Journal of Investigational Allergology and Clinical Immunology*, **5**, 6–11

Reed, C.E. Diagnosing asthma: past, present and future. *Journal of Asthma*, **31**, 327–8

Reilly, D., Taylor, M.A., Beattie, N.G.M. *et al.* Is evidence for homeopathy reproducible? *Lancet*, **244**, 1601–6

Robinson, D.S. and Geddes, D.M. Inhaled corticosteroids: benefits and risks. *Journal of Asthma*, **33**, 5–16

Tilles, S.A. and Nelson, H.S. Long-acting inhaled beta-agonists. *Journal of Asthma*, **32**, 397–404

Tinkelman, D. and Conner, B. Diagnosis and management of asthma in the young child. *Journal of Asthma*, **31**, 419–25

Trigg, C. and Lee, T. Wasp and bee venom immunotherapy. *Asthma Journal*, December 1995, 12–15

Utiger, R.D. Differences between inhaled and oral glucocorticoid therapy. *New England Journal of Medicine*, **329**, 1731–3

Wolthers, O.D. and Pedersen, S. Growth of asthmatic children during treatment with budesonide: a double blind trial. *British Medical Journal*, **303**, 163–5

Wolthers, O.D. and Pedersen, S. Short-term growth during treatment with inhaled fluticasone propionate and beclomethasone diprorionate. *Archives of Disease in Childhood*, **68**, 673–76

Young, E., Stoneham, M.D., Petruckevitch, A. *et al.* A population study of food intolerance. *Lancet*, **343**, 1127–30

Yung, B. and Campbell, I.A. Steroid-induced osteoporosis. *Asthma Journal*, December 1995, 16–19

INDEX